A CONCISE HISTORY
OF EUTHANASIA

Critical Issues in History
Series Editor: Donald T. Critchlow

A CONCISE HISTORY OF EUTHANASIA

Life, Death, God, and Medicine

IAN DOWBIGGIN

ROWMAN & LITTLEFIELD PUBLISHERS, INC.
Lanham • Boulder • New York • Toronto • Plymouth, UK

ROWMAN & LITTLEFIELD PUBLISHERS, INC.

Published in the United States of America
by Rowman & Littlefield Publishers, Inc.
A wholly owned subsidiary of The Rowman & Littlefield Publishing Group, Inc.
4501 Forbes Boulevard, Suite 200, Lanham, Maryland 20706
www.rowmanlittlefield.com

Estover Road, Plymouth PL6 7PY, United Kingdom

Copyright © 2005 by Rowman & Littlefield Publishers, Inc.
First paperback edition 2007.

British Library Cataloguing in Publication Information Available

**The hardback edition of this book was catalogued by the Library of
Congress as follows:**

Dowbiggin, Ian Robert, 1952-
   A concise history of euthanasia : life, death, God, and medicine / Ian Dowbiggin.
      p. cm.— (Critical issues in history)
   Includes bibliographical references and index.
   1. Euthanasia. I. Title. II. Series.
   R726.D688 2005
   179.7—dc22
                                                                        2005001704
ISBN-13: 978-0-7425-3110-9 (cloth : alk. paper)
ISBN-10: 0-7425-3110-4 (cloth : alk. paper)
ISBN-13: 978-0-7425-3111-6 (pbk. : alk. paper)
ISBN-10: 0-7425-3111-2 (pbk. : alk. paper)

Printed in the United States of America

♾™ The paper used in this publication meets the minimum requirements of
American National Standard for Information Sciences—Permanence of Paper for
Printed Library Materials, ANSI/NISO Z39.48-1992.

CONTENTS

v

ACKNOWLEDGMENTS

I wish to thank the Social Sciences and Humanities Research Council of Canada and the University of Prince Edward Island for their generous support of the research that made this book possible. I have also benefited immeasurably from conversations with Keith Cassidy, Donald Critchlow, Derek Jeffrey, Edward Larson, Daryl Pullman, Susan McEachern, Doug Payne, Christine Rosen, Alex Schadenberg, William Seidelman, Wesley Smith, Richard Weikart, and Kevin Yuill. While few of them would agree with all the conclusions I reach, all have helped to make this book better.

INTRODUCTION:
A QUESTION OF VALUES

On January 7, 1998, in a hushed Toronto courtroom, Mark Jewitt sat and watched history being made. In the same courtroom, the fifty-one-year-old Maurice Genereux, Jewitt's former doctor, became the first physician in North American history ever convicted of assisted suicide. Two months later, Genereux was stripped of his license to practice medicine by a disciplinary committee of Ontario's College of Physicians and Surgeons. On May 13, 1998, Genereux was sent to jail for two years less a day, a sentence that was upheld on appeal a year later.

As he intently viewed the courtroom proceedings, the thought must have crossed Jewitt's mind that he was lucky to be alive. Two and a half years earlier, Jewitt had been profoundly depressed over the death of his male lover from acquired immune deficiency syndrome (AIDS). Haunted by his own HIV-positive diagnosis, Jewitt had asked Genereux to prescribe him fifty pills of Seconal, a powerful barbiturate and popular suicide drug in the city's gay community. When Jewitt came close to overdosing and lapsed into a coma, a friend saved him by calling 911.

Aaron McGinn, another Genereux patient, was not so lucky. McGinn, like Jewitt, young, gay, and in good physical health, succeeded in committing suicide in 1996 after ingesting an overdose of the sleeping pills that Genereux had prescribed. Genereux then falsified McGinn's death certificate to make it appear that he had died from AIDS. But a Toronto psychiatrist familiar with McGinn's emotional troubles reported his suspicions to the city's chief coroner, who started an investigation that culminated in Genereux's arrest on June 20, 1996.

As he counted his blessings that day in early 1998, Jewitt likely did not realize that the events unfolding before him were another powerful historical reminder of how euthanasia had become one of the most controversial and

1

significant health-care issues at the beginning of the new millennium. Few moments in history better dramatized the myriad new and long-standing aspects of euthanasia. The term "euthanasia" comes from the Greek word for "good death" and was first coined by the English philosopher Francis Bacon in the early seventeenth century. Death is the grim equalizer. While few people will die the same way as Aaron McGinn, sooner or later everyone will share his ultimate fate. Thus, how society defines what is and is not a good death potentially affects every human being. It is the haunting question that lies at the heart of the evolving history of euthanasia.

History demonstrates that euthanasia has meant different things to people at different times throughout the past. Today, it can mean Maurice Genereux's crime, providing patients with pills or other methods to end their lives, the act of assisting suicide. Or euthanasia can mean what Jack Kevorkian, the notorious "Doctor Death," did to fifty-two-year-old Thomas Youk as documented on the CBS *60 Minutes* news program on November 22, 1998. Kevorkian injected poison into Youk, who was suffering from amyotrophic lateral sclerosis, or Lou Gehrig's disease. Before killing Youk, Kevorkian had already helped ninety-three other individuals to die between 1990 and 1998. A court later found him guilty of murdering Youk, sentencing him to ten years' imprisonment. Kevorkian hastened Youk's death, an act of active euthanasia and a crime in every American state and all countries around the world, except the Netherlands. Nonetheless, Kevorkian has many admirers, including *60 Minutes* host Mike Wallace.

Euthanasia can also mean the withdrawal of life-sustaining treatment for chronically ill persons, which happened to Terri Schiavo of Clearwater, Florida. In 1990, Schiavo collapsed from cardiac arrest at the age of twenty-six and lapsed into a coma-like state. Thanks to a medical malpractice ruling, a court awarded her husband, Michael Schiavo, $750,000 for Terri's rehabilitation. Michael had a "do not resuscitate" order placed on her chart, claiming this is what Terri would have wanted. In 1998, Michael went to court again, this time to have Terri's food and fluids discontinued. A judge's decision to allow Terri's death by starvation and dehydration launched a case that ended in 2005 when Terri died after her feeding tube was removed. The legal wrangle pitted Michael Schiavo against Terri's parents, who insisted she could be revived through rehabilitation.

What happened to Terri Schiavo takes place routinely in hospices, hospitals, and nursing homes throughout the world, even though death by starvation and dehydration is a painful, drawn-out process. Though often considered merciful, it is anything but a good death.

The Terri Schiavo, Maurice Genereux, and Jack Kevorkian stories bring the history of euthanasia up to date in vivid, human ways. They reveal that acts of euthanasia are not infrequent, isolated incidents. Some of these acts are done in accordance with patients' prior wishes. Often they are done when patients' genuine wishes are not at all clear. Typically, a host of motives surrounds an act of euthanasia. Compassion and a deep respect for human rights frequently co-exist with concerns about the rising costs of health care or the convenience of family and friends. Jewitt's encounter with Maurice Genereux, like so many other episodes in the history of euthanasia, reveals that it is rarely easy to disentangle the different motives behind a single act of euthanasia. Whatever the motives, however, the result is all too often human tragedy.

Genereux's actions were indicative of how common euthanasia practices are today. His medical career, punctuated by personal drug, alcohol, and sexual misconduct problems, should have been a warning to others that he was not equipped to treat seriously ill and emotionally vulnerable patients. Two years before he was charged with assisting suicide, he had been convicted by the provincial College of Physicians and Surgeons for fondling six different male patients. He was never disciplined. The medical community feared that Genereux's removal would further deplete the city's undersupply of doctors willing to minister to patients afflicted with AIDS. But, as events proved, the trade-off was one sided. Genereux was little more than a "scrip doctor," in Mark Jewitt's words, a "Pez dispenser" for narcotics and sleeping pills, willing to write prescriptions to depressed HIV-positive men who dreaded dying of AIDS.

Genereux's defenders claimed he was simply responding to the demand for his services, and in one sense that is true. A major thrust behind the campaign in the early twenty-first century to legalize physician-assisted suicide in Canada and elsewhere comes from those who disproportionately suffer from AIDS-related illnesses. As AIDS cut its lethal swath through the world's homosexual communities in the 1980s and 1990s, it helped to energize what had come to be called the right-to-die movement, the efforts of groups seeking the legalization of active euthanasia and physician-assisted suicide. It is not difficult to see why. AIDS patients normally die "hard deaths." As the human immunodeficiency virus insidiously invades and kills the body's immune cells, various microbes and cancers attack the body's organ systems. This can leave the patient demented, starving, bleeding internally, unable to breathe, or ravaged by tumors. Medical technology designed to keep patients alive, developed since the mid-twentieth century, prolongs the suffering of AIDS patients, until they are little more than disfigured, shriveled specimens of the young, active individuals they had once been. AIDS is a painful and macabre way to die, and those with the condition know it, hence the large percentage of suicides, assisted or otherwise, among the AIDS population. Despite recent improvements in treatment, an AIDS diagnosis strikes many as a virtual death sentence few sadists could imagine. Little wonder that AIDS patients sought out Genereux.

Genereux's activities revealed that there was a euthanasia "underground" in Toronto's gay community, a network of doctors who were willing to provide AIDS patients with the narcotics to kill themselves and then to write death certificates that covered up their crimes. Toronto's gay village resembles other homosexual communities around the world, such as that of the San Francisco Bay area, where almost half of the doctors who treated HIV-infected patients confessed to assisting at least one suicide of an AIDS patient in the mid-1990s. Research indicates that when a physician is gay himself, as was Genereux, he may have difficulty being objective in the face of an impassioned appeal from a patient whose sexual orientation is the same.[1]

Ultimately, Genereux ended up in court, not because the legal system ordinarily catches similar acts of assisted suicide, but because he was clumsy and did little to hide what he was doing. The crucial question is: how many people such as Jewitt and McGinn were simply depressed and yet had their requests for assisted suicide honored by a sympathetic physician? Jewitt certainly believed Genereux had failed as a physician by acceding to his request and doing virtually nothing to change his mind. Jewitt testified against Genereux in court and later launched civil proceedings against him. There is no way of knowing whether Jewitt was typical of the many men in his situation, but it is clear that he was grateful to have a second lease on life. His treatment at the hands of Genereux is a chilling reminder that determining whether a patient really wants to die is anything but straightforward.

How did history arrive at the events that so tragically affected the lives of Mark Jewitt and Aaron McGinn? As this book demonstrates, the fates of Jewitt and McGinn were the products of a long and dramatic history. It is a history that inevitably encompasses shifting patterns in mortality due to disease and disability. Conditions such as AIDS, Alzheimer's disease, and the various types of cancer indicate that many people will endure protracted, painful, and undignified deaths.

The history of euthanasia is also a story that is influenced by technological and behavioral changes in the practice of medicine. Today, when modern medicine can do so much to prolong lives, it is no coincidence that a right-to-die movement flourishes in many countries around the world.

The specter of being kept alive through artificial means terrifies numerous people into supporting legislation that gives them the power to choose the time, manner, and place of their deaths.

Yet, even more importantly, as this book argues, the history of euthanasia has been largely conditioned by evolving opinions about what constitutes a good death, which in turn has depended on shifting value systems governing such things as sin, suffering, resignation, judgment, penance, and redemption. In the last century or so, the debate over euthanasia has broken down into a bitter struggle between two formidable groups. On one side are those who try to reconcile the changing technical landscape of modern medicine with the traditional moral values that defend the sanctity of individual human life. Rather than a right to die, they stress a right to compassionate and effective end-of-life care. At the turn of the twenty-first century, this is the spirit of the World Health Organization's recommendation that governments not consider legalizing assisted suicide or active euthanasia until they have ensured that high-quality palliative care is available to all their citizens. This is also the spirit of Pope John Paul II's 2004 statement that food and water should never be withheld from patients such as Terri Schiavo, whose own end-of-life wishes have never been obvious.

On the other side of the debate are those who seek to interpret the worth of human life in terms of either biological criteria, utilitarian standards, a faith in science, humane medical treatment, the principle of personal autonomy, or individual human rights. These views of human life date back far beyond the revolutionary inception of sophisticated medical machinery for prolonging life to earlier turning points in the history of Western civilization, such as the eighteenth-century Enlightenment and the coming of Darwinism in the late nineteenth century. That the arguments of euthanasia advocates grew more plausible than ever before at a time when technological innovations first made their mark is undeniable. But the theory that they were *determined* by such changes does not fit the historical facts. At bottom, what has tended to unite the movement in favor of legal euthanasia, at least in Western cultures, has been an eagerness to challenge traditional Judeo-Christian approaches to the morality of suicide and mercy killing.

Victory in this struggle over euthanasia as the twenty-first century dawns ultimately depends on the specific national contexts in which it takes place. Countries with dissimilar political cultures will frequently differ over how to define the good death. The stakes include who gets to say what it means to treat the sick, disabled, and dying with compassion, respect, generosity, and justice. The chronically and terminally ill as well as persons with disabilities, young and old, are people whose human rights entitle them to make decisions about their own lives. Yet they also rely heavily on the merciful intentions of family, friends, and caregivers. Ultimately, everyone dies "in the arms of others," to one extent or another.[2] The history of twentieth-century euthanasia provides us with plenty of evidence of what can happen when a community is willing to rank the individual lives of vulnerable people in terms of happiness, pleasure, dignity, social usefulness, or economic productivity. The past confirms that a "moral free fall," to quote bioethicist Wesley Smith, is indeed a distinct danger in the early twenty-first century.[3]

The final chapter in the history of euthanasia remains to be written. But if this history reveals anything to date, it is that the many issues surrounding death, dying, suicide, disease, palliative care, and terminal illness deserve more debate. As the U.S. physician and award-winning author Sherwin Nuland has argued persuasively, death still needs to be demythologized.[4] Until the twentieth century, people were frequent witnesses to the reality of death. Men, women, and children saw death in its many forms, and they constructed rituals and codes of conduct to explain how, why, and when it struck. By contrast, in the twenty-first century, there appears to be a troubling silence surrounding aging and death. The public remains strangely unaware of death's many clinical and biological dimensions. Nuland is right: educating the public on these dimensions can reduce the persistent fears many feel when their own deaths or the deaths of others are imminent. These fears, once muted by the consolations of religious belief, are what primarily drive the demand for euthanasia. The history of euthanasia in the twenty-first century hinges on whether the nations of the world can conquer these fears and take the policy steps to ensure that in future no one has to suffer like Mark Jewitt.

NOTES

1. Lee R. Slome et al., "Physician-Assisted Suicide and Patients with Human Immunodeficiency Virus Disease," *New England Journal of Medicine* 336, no. 6 (1997): 417–421.

2. Peter G. Filene, *In the Arms of Others: A Cultural History of the Right-to-Die in America* (Chicago: Ivan Dee, 1998).

3. Wesley J. Smith, *Forced Exit: The Slippery Slope from Assisted Suicide to Legalized Murder* (New York: Random House, 1997).

4. Sherwin B. Nuland, *How We Die: Reflections on Life's Final Chapter* (New York: Knopf, 1994), xvi–xvii.

1

OBEDIENT UNTO DEATH

The story is told by Pliny the Younger (62–114 AD), the renowned Roman writer, lawyer, orator, and administrator. Sketchy in detail, the tale nonetheless says a great deal about the nonjudgmental attitude of the ancient Romans toward the question of what constituted a "good death." Much later, in the twentieth century, some euthanasia advocates would look back fondly on this viewpoint and cite it as a reason for overturning accepted interpretations of the value of human life. But in the short term, the ancient Roman definition of a good death was toppled by the revolutionary Christian doctrine upholding the sanctity of life and condemning anything that resembled suicide, assisted suicide, or mercy killing. This doctrine about the equal value of all human lives would reign largely unchallenged until the eighteenth-century Enlightenment.

SUICIDE IN CLASSICAL ANTIQUITY

As Pliny the Younger told the story, a certain man was suffering from an unspecified disease of the genital organs. His wife asked to see the affected part. Having satisfied her curiosity, she promptly declared his condition to be incurable and deadly. Her advice was that the couple should jointly commit suicide by drowning, though there is no indication that the husband ardently shared her opinion. Whatever his intentions, they ended up throwing themselves into a lake together.

This story of a suicide pact between a husband and wife is only one of many tales of suicide in classical antiquity. Many ancient Greek and Roman philosophers considered suicide a "good death," an appropriate and rational response to a wide variety of circumstances. There are numerous accounts of people killing themselves by poison, fasting, asphyxiation, hanging, or slitting their wrists. Motives ran the gamut from pains due to cancer, bladder stones, stomach disorders, gout, and headaches, to melancholy, the fear of dishonor, and the hope of avoiding judgment and execution. Individuals frequently asked their physicians to either supply them with the means of suicide (assisted suicide) or actually hasten their deaths through medical intervention (active voluntary euthanasia), for example by administering poison. Quite simply, assisting suicide and mercy killing were common and tolerated practices in ancient Greece and early imperial Rome.[1]

Suicide and euthanasia were common acts in classical antiquity because fundamentally they did not conflict with the moral beliefs of the time. The ancients were fairly permissive about self-murder and euthanasia. In stark contrast to the teaching of most modern-day Christian churches, Jewish religious bodies, and other world religions, the ancient Greeks and Romans did not think that all human life had an inherent value. They tended to reject any semblance of the belief in the sanctity of human life, or the modern notion that all people enjoyed a range of natural rights by virtue of a universal property of their human condition. When faced with hopeless circumstances, the ancient Greeks and Romans suffered little social disapproval if they chose to end their lives, commit infanticide, or perform abortions.

Actual attitudes toward suicide were far from uniform in ancient Greece. The Epicureans and Pythagorean schools of philosophy condemned it as a rebellion against the will of God. However, many other thinkers, such as Plato, praised it as noble and heroic if it avoided dishonor or the agony of a long terminal illness. The Stoics tended to agree, inspiring many of the best-known suicides in classical antiquity, such as Cato the Elder (234–149 BC). The Stoics regarded the taking of one's own life as a perfectly rational response to specific situations. The ancient Greek philosopher Aristotle may have taken a dim view of suicide, but his reasoning (that the suicide was denying the state the duties owed it by a citizen) had nothing to do with any concept of the sanctity of life.

The example of Sparta graphically demonstrates to what extremes the ancient Greek toleration of suicide and euthanasia could lead. Sparta, which inspired Plato's theory of an ideal state, was based on a value system that stressed breeding and training the most vigorous citizens possible. Infants deemed "feeble and ill-shaped," the Greek historian Plutarch (46–120 AD) tells us, were put to death in Sparta. Invalids of all ages were allowed to die. Strictly speaking, this was not euthanasia, since the method of death was rarely painless and sometimes cruel. But the Spartans believed that, for all concerned, a person ill-suited for health and service to the state was better off dead than alive. Even in Athens, Sparta's arch-foe among the Greek city-states, the regular form of punishment was self-destruction.

As far as the ancient Romans were concerned, suicide was legally permitted, except for slaves, criminals, and soldiers. It was frequently viewed as a triumph over fate. The Roman scholar Pliny the Elder (23–79 AD) was convinced that the ability to commit suicide was "the greatest advantage" God had given humankind.[2] To Pliny, the freedom to kill oneself was a sign of one's autonomy and one's power over the vagaries of existence. The philosopher Seneca insisted that choosing suicide at the appropriate time was a basic individual right. Seneca, who committed suicide in 65 AD when implicated in a conspiracy against the emperor Nero, went beyond earlier justifications of suicide in imperial Rome that cited dishonor or suffering. He instead celebrated suicide as a valuable and handy means for exiting the world. Later nineteenth- and twentieth-century support for legalizing euthanasia sometimes echoed this view that suicide might not be a remedy for all of life's ills, but it was available to the rational, educated, and adult human being who was convinced there was no reason to live anymore.

The willingness of some ancient Greek and Roman writers to ascribe a positive value to suicide or mercy killing signaled a significant break with the customs of other civilized communities of much earlier times. Infanticide, abortion, and suicide were common occurrences in most if not all aboriginal societies from the South Seas to the tundras of the Arctic. Yet abandonment or exposure of infants and the elderly were chiefly motivated by grim concerns about available food supply and the survival prospects of the clan or tribe, not by any abstract belief that death was preferable to life when sickness or disability occurred. The murder of disabled or inconvenient individuals was balanced by a natural love of life and an impressive fondness for children and other family members. If aboriginal societies tolerated what in retrospect looks like cruel acts, it was simply because of the demands of the community trying to eke out a meager existence in an unforgiving natural environment.

The attitudes, if not the practices, of aboriginal societies stood in sharp contrast to the opinions of the ancient Greeks and Romans. The ancient Greek and Roman approach to euthanasia stemmed to a large extent from the state of health care and the nature of the medical profession in classical antiquity. There is every indication that Greeks and Romans in antiquity faced few problems finding physicians to provide them with assistance in dying. No system of medical licensure existed, nor were any professional standards enforceable by law or medical organizations, as has been the case over the last century or so. Rival schools of medicine abounded and engaged in heated polemics. Healers were relatively free to practice their craft as they saw fit.

However, this kind of free market in medicine came with a price for physicians. Without the legitimacy provided by professional organization, state-authorized licensing, and educational credentialism, physicians did not enjoy the type of respect they were to enjoy in the modern era. The Romans tended to regard their physicians with contempt, because most of them were slaves or Greeks. Romans expected their physicians to carry out orders, even if it meant helping their patrons end their lives. Most doctors in antiquity in any case were reluctant to take on incurable cases, leaving terminally ill patients with few medical options other than euthanasia. In all probability, the majority of requests for euthanasia or assisted suicide were fulfilled in classical antiquity.

As much as some modern-day supporters of euthanasia might look back on this state of affairs as desirable, it had an undeniably cautionary side. Pliny the Younger's tale of the suicide pact, sketchy as it is, raises numerous questions about suicide and euthanasia both today and two millennia ago. How mentally balanced was the wife in trying to talk her husband into killing themselves? Did she simply refuse to live without her husband? Obviously a trusting soul, her husband took her word that he was destined to die soon, without consulting a qualified physician. Was he too despondent or foolish to seek other advice? Was he talked into suicide by the woman he loved, or was he instead afraid of a lingering, painful death? The absence of firm answers to these questions suggests strongly that there were psychiatric dimensions to this joint suicide, enough to alarm even the most casual of observers.

THE HIPPOCRATIC OATH

Perhaps the most important aspect of the story told by Pliny the Younger is that he offered no moral opinion about the act of suicide. His suspension of judgment indicates that such events were fairly routine and often drew little comment. If Pliny's opinions about suicide were in any way indicative of reality, they help to explain why the Hippocratic Oath forbade the participation of physicians in acts designed to shorten the lives of patients. Little is known precisely about the oath's origins, but it is generally thought to be the product of more than one solitary physician called Hippocrates and to date from between the fifth and third centuries BC. Before the Christian era, it did not draw much attention from physicians or other people. Its value as a historical document is that it sheds light on what likely passed for customary medical practice.[3]

Among its several injunctions is the first clear denunciation of mercy killing or assisted suicide in Western medical history. The Hippocratic body of writings contains several references encouraging physicians to refrain from life-prolonging treatment if the patient is dying. The oath also reads: "I will not give a fatal drug to anyone if I am asked, nor will I suggest any such thing." The oath's authority has resonated down through the ages to the present day, when physicians swear to the god Apollo to keep the oath to the best of their "ability and judgment." The Hippocratic Oath is a milestone in the history of medicine because it articulated the lofty goals of the selfless doctor who would inspire later generations of physicians, a model of professional competence and probity. It also strongly expressed the theory that physicians should look for the causes of and remedies for disease in purely natural explanations of sickness.[4] But the oath's blanket prohibition against euthanasia (and abortion) has met increasing resistance in recent years.

Two things can be said about the oath with some assurance: first, many ancient Greek and Roman physicians did not abide by its injunctions, and second, the oath's prohibition of euthanasia plainly was a kind of protest against the frequency with which euthanasia was practiced in the years before the revolutionary coming of Christianity. There never would have been a need for the oath's injunction if euthanasia had been rare in the first place. The oath's influence became powerful only in later centuries. In the meantime, it confirmed the prevailing belief in classical antiquity that there was nothing inconsistent between the values of that day and physician-assisted suicide or actual medical mercy killing.

JUDAISM

The attitude of ancient Romans and Greeks in favor of medical assistance in dying steadily met resistance in the first centuries of the common era, thanks to two formidable forces in world history. The first was Judaism. In the words of the Central Conference of American Rabbis in 1972, "the Jewish ideal of the sanctity of human life and the supreme value of the individual soul would suffer incalculable harm if, contrary to the moral law, men were at liberty to determine the conditions under which they might put an end to their own lives and the lives of other men." As late as 1997, even Reform Judaism, the most liberal of all branches of Judaism, refused to declare that euthanasia was consistent with Jewish values.[5]

The reasons for the firm Jewish religious opposition to both assisted suicide and mercy killing are sprinkled throughout the Jewish scriptures, which constitute the Christian Old Testament. On multiple occasions in the Old Testament, God is acknowledged to exercise an absolute sovereignty over life and death. Death was the penalty for sin, and life was a gift from God that his people were meant to choose so they could continue to love, honor, and obey him. Choosing death was an affront to God that demonstrated contempt for the gift of life: "No man has authority . . . over the day of death" (Ecclesiastes 8:8). The scriptures contain some examples of Jews willingly dying as martyrs or choosing suicide, but they do so because they prefer death to violating Judaic law. And none of these examples occurs in conditions remotely resembling the circumstances surrounding modern-day medical euthanasia or physician-assisted suicide. Throughout the Old Testament, there is no instance of Jews either killing themselves or arranging for someone else to help them die due to the physical anguish of illness.

These firm Jewish beliefs about suicide and euthanasia spread throughout the Roman imperial world thanks to the huge Jewish diaspora. Even before the catastrophe of 66–70 AD, when a large-scale Jewish revolt was crushed mercilessly by the Romans and the Temple in Jerusalem was destroyed by the imperial armies, the Jews were a powerful presence throughout the Mediterranean region. Sizeable communities could be found in cities such as Alexandria, Antioch, Damascus, and even Rome itself. Jewish value systems probably had little effect on pagan Romans. But when they became synthesized with the beliefs of the growing numbers of Christian converts sprinkled throughout the Roman Empire, they steadily shaped public attitudes as the new millennium wore on.

THE COMING OF CHRISTIANITY

The emergence of Christianity in the first century AD was the other momentous factor that shaped the new era in the history of euthanasia. Basic Christian values about death and dying are similar to the Judaic moral code, although explicit condemnations of suicide are missing from the New Testament. It was in later centuries that the church fathers inferred from the Gospels that suicide was against God's law. A major spokesperson for this theory was Saint Augustine (354–430 AD), who in his *City of God* (428) argued that suicide was simply another form of homicide, and thus was both a crime and a sin prohibited by the sixth of the Ten Commandments. In Augustine's eyes, even those who opted for suicide in order to avoid a sin (such as a virgin seeking to protect her virtue) were actually committing a greater sin and forfeited the possibility of repentance.

The fact that the word "suicide" was coined much later in history (the seventeenth century) to replace the phrase "self-murder" signifies that for centuries Christians followed Augustine's thinking and regarded the taking of one's own life as a form of murder, and thus an abhorrent crime that required no formal condemnation. This was true even in cases of martyrdom when Christians went willingly to their deaths at the hands of imperial authorities. Undoubtedly, some early Christians provoked martyrdom, a thinly veiled form of suicide. Theologians such as Clement of Alexandria (150–215 AD) tried to discourage overeager martyrs by distinguishing between aggressive attempts to achieve death by persecution and dying for one's faith. But before the legalization of Christianity in 313 AD, throughout the empire the consensus among Christians was that martyrdom was a glorious fate to submit to, and as such had nothing to do with taking one's life by one's own hands. Martyrdom testified to an individual's faith and was distinguished from suicide undertaken for nonreligious motives.

Clement's uneasiness about where a thirst for martyrdom might lead was confirmed later in history when whole communities sometimes chose suicide on a mass scale. Twelfth-century Cathars and Albigensians, declared heretics by the medieval church, were renowned for their willingness to kill themselves in the pursuit of what they imagined was the holy life rather than abjure their faith. Much later, "Old Believers" in Russia resisted attempts to modernize Eastern Orthodox Christianity. Some locked themselves in monasteries in the late seventeenth century and burned them to the ground, perishing in the flames, rather than submit to liturgical changes. Other religious dissenters in late nineteenth-century Russia buried themselves alive in order to escape census taking, which they regarded as sinful. These shocking examples of self-destruction help to explain why Christian churches traditionally have opposed either religious or secular attempts to approve of suicide.

The same attitude applies to Christian asceticism, the mortification of the flesh that was often practiced by the early monks and other Christians. Some Christians, in their pursuit of a more intense and personal union with God, and once opportunities for martyrdom vanished with the official toleration of Christianity in the fourth century, punished themselves physically by rigorous fasting and exposure to the elements of nature.

Yet, the New Testament did not advocate any self-discipline that might lead to death. If strict asceticism led to death, Christian theologians argued, the crucial question was whether or not the ascetic intended to kill himself.

If not, it was not suicide, and hence not a sin. This was an early variation of the later, twentieth-century theory of a "double effect" in euthanasia, which stated that a physician whose painkillers led to a patient's death was not guilty of medical murder if the physician had administered the drugs in the sincere hopes of merely mitigating anguish rather than producing euthanasia. In other words, a valid distinction can be drawn between consequences that are intended and those that are foreseen (and even inevitable) but not desired.

All in all, then, in the early centuries of the new millennium, the attitude of Christians toward life and death was that human beings inhabited a fallen world in which suffering had to be endured as the penalty of sin. The life we enjoy is a gift from God, who remains sovereign over all things, and any effort to end existence through suicide or aid in dying is a shameful attempt to escape the trials that God in his wisdom has decided to inflict or permit. Allowances sometimes were made for suicides during a state of mental illness. But, in the end analysis, Christians were taught to be "obedient unto death," in Saint Paul's words (see Philippians 2:5–11). Suffering emulated the suffering of Christ and provided human beings with an opportunity to sanctify their lives.

OTHER WORLD RELIGIONS

In overturning ancient Greek and Roman ethics about death and dying, Christianity was echoing what other major world religions basically decreed about suicide. Just as the distinctions between suicide and martyrdom were sometimes murky in Christianity, religions such as Hinduism—though generally hostile toward suicide for nonreligious reasons—praised self-sacrifice that culminated in death. Holy persons who renounced the world and starved themselves to death to achieve freedom from all desires were respected. Likewise, the practice of sati, in which a widow climbed the funeral pyre of her deceased husband to join him in death, survived for centuries until it was outlawed by the British in 1829. However, aside from examples of ascetic religious suicide, sati remained the exception in Hinduism, which heavily censures ordinary forms of self-murder. Sikhism, too, does not permit suicide. The belief in reincarnation and the absolute acceptance of God's will deters Sikhs from taking their own lives, requesting assistance in suicide, or outright mercy killing.

Buddhism also forbids suicide because it violates the first of five fundamental precepts: "kill not any living thing." The Buddha appears to have disapproved of suicide. According to Buddhist teaching, human beings are expected to live their allotted spans of life. Voluntary death is not considered an acceptable means of avoiding sufferings that are due to former deeds. "Where there is life, there is hope," Buddhism teaches. For Buddhists, euthanasia is based on a materialist view of life, and while it might end the suffering of loved ones, it cannot end the kharma of suffering that persists in the dead patient.[6] The rule is that suicide is generally forbidden for the vast majority of believers. In Confucianism, persons who commit suicide rob their ancestors of the veneration and service due to them and demonstrate ingratitude to parents for the gift of life.

The arrival of Islam in the seventh century, despite defying Christianity and Judaism in many other respects, did not challenge Christian and Judaic teaching about suicide. Controversy surrounds the question of whether the Koran specifically forbids suicide, but there is general agreement that the prophet Muhammad intended to prohibit self-murder. Martyrs who die defending their faith are highly commended in Islam and are rewarded by immediate entrance into paradise, where they will enjoy great sensual pleasures. But virtually all forms of suicide are strongly condemned. Islamic teaching says that those who kill themselves are denied paradise and sentenced to hell, where they must spend their time repeating the act that ended their lives. Like Christianity, Islam draws a solid distinction between religiously motivated martyrdom and the act of self-destruction to escape the trials and tribulations of life. To Islam, modern-day suicide bombers are martyrs for their faith, not suicides in the sense of people who kill themselves because they find life intolerable. In Islam, as in Christianity, suicide was both a sin and crime for centuries down to the modern era.

The persistence and prevalence of these beliefs about suicide today signifies that euthanasia is even more foreign a practice to the Muslim than to the Christian mind. In Islamic thought, pain and suffering are the price believers pay for sin. Euthanasia therefore constitutes an interference with expiation for sin, and thus subverts the divine plan.

The crucial point is that up to the twentieth century, although all the major world religions recognized certain instances in which voluntary death was permissible, they nonetheless were unanimous in condemning those who killed themselves or others in order to relieve misery. The willingness to die for one's faith, or sacrifice oneself to a deity as a means of renouncing material desires, is so alien to modern-day justifications of the right to die that there is really no meaningful comparison. The exceptions that have been made for self-sacrifice for religious motives simply prove the rule that none of the major world religions sanctions ending a life to cut short the anguish caused by disease or dying.

SUICIDE IN THE MIDDLE AGES

After the collapse of the Roman Empire, and as the Middle Ages unfolded over the next one thousand years, any semblance of ancient approval for suicide or mercy killing vanished throughout the Western world. The Christian view that suicide was a serious sin and major crime took root steadily, and it ultimately became so accepted in the medieval mind that there existed virtually no debate over the subject. The anti-suicide consensus was reflected in clerical doctrine and secular literature and law. Any doubts about the acceptability of suicide were erased during the medieval era by the spectacle of the severe punishments meted out to the bodies of suicides and their surviving families.

The Augustinian viewpoint that suicide was nothing less than murder dominated medieval discussions of the topic. Theologians such as Abelard, Duns Scotus, John of Salisbury, and Jean Buridan argued that in no case was it religiously permissible to take one's own life. Thomas Aquinas (c. 1225–1274), the most influential of medieval theologians, subjected the justifications for suicide to rigorous analysis and rejected them all. Suicide deprived society of the roles we are expected to play; it defied the natural instinct to live and the duty to love ourselves; it offended God, the proprietor of all life. Aquinas concluded that "whoever takes his own life, sins against God." Death was the most important moment of an individual's life, the time for Christians to prepare their souls to meet their divine master. Clergy were expected to be there to perform the sacraments, console the dying, and enable them to confess. The idea that in such a setting one might request another to help one commit suicide was strictly forbidden in Thomist philosophy. So authoritative were Aquinas's teachings on suicide that their echoes were still evident in the Vatican's 1980 declaration against assisted dying.

Secular literature in the medieval period tended to be as hostile to suicide as official religious teaching. Popular drama condemned suicide as vigorously as the most orthodox theologian. Some *chansons de geste*, such as the twelfth-century ballad *The Song of Roland*, contained examples of Christian warrior knights fighting gloriously but hopelessly to the death, when they could have saved themselves by retreating or requesting reinforcements. Yet these deaths were examples of knights trying to live up to the chivalric code of honor and bravery, and when other characters killed themselves out of shame, sorrow, or pain, it was regarded as a sign of personal failure and sin, no matter how extenuating the circumstances. In courtly literature, instances abound of heroes and heroines killing themselves, but here, too, the abundantly clear message is that they do so because it is the lesser of two evils. The medieval view was summed up by the great Italian poet Dante Alighieri (1265–1321). In Dante's *Inferno* (1313–1321), there is a special place for suicides in the seventh circle of hell, devoid of all human form and tormented by harpies for all eternity.

Canon and civil law, with their severe penalties for suicide, upheld the medieval consensus that self-murder was a terrible crime and sin. Public demonstrations of this consensus served as graphic reminders that taking one's own life was strictly forbidden. For example, when one man in Paris in the thirteenth century killed himself and the local abbey had the man's body hanged, a royal official ordered that the execution be repeated, with the corpse first being dragged through the streets. In other instances, the corpse of a suicide could be denied burial in consecrated ground, or the estate of the deceased could be confiscated. Some localities ordered the body of a suicide to be nailed to a barrel and cast into the river to be carried far away by the current. Such fates awaited other suicides unless magistrates or clergy could be persuaded that those who killed themselves were mentally ill.[7] Yet, even when those in authority agreed that madness was the cause, the act itself remained staunchly forbidden.

Of course, the fierce medieval prohibition against suicide did not mean the practice was nonexistent. Throughout the Middle Ages, for example, peasants and craftspeople hanged themselves to escape humiliation or painful suffering. Monks in fits of solitary despair threw themselves out of the windows of high towers. Knights banished from their ladies' sight chose their swords to end their own lives. The taboo against suicide never eliminated the act entirely.

Still, the taboo's influence was far reaching and powerful. When confronted with the fact that suicide never disappeared, medieval Europeans increasingly attributed the practice to either insanity or possession by the devil. It was thought that no suicides could be in their right minds. When insanity or possession was the consensus of opinion in a particular case, the usual punishments were normally waived.

MEDIEVAL MEDICINE

The medieval age also witnessed a distinct change in the practice of medicine, a shift that further undercut the ancient permissiveness toward suicide and euthanasia. In antiquity, physicians were not expected to have anything to do with the dying. The main task of ancient Greek and Roman doctors was to cure patients, and if a case was deemed to be hopeless, the attending physician who stayed with the terminally ill patient was most often suspected of mercenary motives. However, as the influence of Christianity spread during the early Middle Ages, physicians began to feel the moral obligation to care for as well as cure patients. The ancient medical code gave way to a new ethos that stressed compassion for the poor, the widow, the orphan, and the sick, resulting in the creation of the first Western hospitals. Medieval hospitals were founded as religious institutions, and within their walls "the Christian ethos was all-pervasive," in the words of medical historian Roy Porter.[8]

By the twelfth and thirteenth centuries, this trend was reinforced by the powerful teachings of moral theologians and the growing professionalization of medicine, which increasingly emphasized the duty of physicians to stay with patients to the bitter end, both comforting the gravely sick and combating their infirmities with all the means at their disposal. As educational and licensing standards for medicine rose, and the network of guilds spread, physicians pledged to treat all in need of medical attention in exchange for a state-guaranteed monopoly for their services.

At the same time, healers became part of a growing custom that united doctor, priest, and family in a deathbed ceremony designed to prepare the terminally ill for their passage from one world to the next. While the physician was present to provide physical comfort, a drama was expected to unfold culminating in what Christians hoped would be a "good death." The good death would involve the administration of the sacraments and provide the opportunity for the sick person to atone for any wrongdoings committed in life. Those in pain, distress, and despair were meant to be comforted in all physical and moral ways, but suffering was also viewed as punishment for past sins and a means of emulating the passion of the Savior himself. "Sickness . . . is that agony in which men are tried for a crown," wrote Jeremy Taylor, a seventeenth-century English Anglican bishop. Taylor's words indicated that the Christian notion of the redemptive power of physical suffering in death persisted long after the waning of the Middle Ages.[9]

The aim of dying well was strongly articulated in the vast body of devotional literature known as the *ars moriendi*. This literary current gathered momentum in the late medieval era and flourished down to the eighteenth century. These were years punctuated by fearsome violence in the form of dynastic conflicts and the religious wars of the Protestant Reformation and Catholic Counter-Reformation. Pestilence, such as bubonic plague and syphilis, spread across the European landscape. Severe want due to poor harvests lurked constantly, bolstering the perception that death lingered over life at every minute. The *ars moriendi* stressed that the ever-presence of death dictated regular and frequent prayer and a continual meditation on human mortality that would only truly make sense in the last hours of life. "He that would die well," wrote British theologian Jeremy Taylor, "must always look for death, every day knocking at the gates of the grave."[10] The tribulations of death, when imminent, were more to be accepted stoically than avoided through aggressive human intervention.

In the midst of the elaborate and deeply emotional drama surrounding death, the physician was forbidden to do anything that might detract from the spiritual journey the patient was undertaking. Any medical hastening of the dying process was strictly prohibited. However, there is no evidence physicians objected. Because they were so limited in their therapeutic power anyway, they tended to embrace their role as bedside participant in the ceremony surrounding a Christian "good death." Whatever their individual religious convictions, they knew that concern for the patient's personal life and general well-being signaled an important part of their fundamental contribution to the death-bed ritual.

Out of this process emerged the modern medical approach to illness, disability, and death, until challenged by the rapid changes of the late twentieth century. In the eyes of society, the church, and their profession, doctors assumed the responsibility of ministering to the sick. They were expected to comfort and console the dying and their loved ones. There was the perpetual tendency for the terminally ill to ignore their spiritual requirements and rely on what treatment a doctor could dispense, to prefer medicine to God. This tension between physical healers and religious authorities festered for centuries, but as long as the therapeutic powers and social standing of organized medicine remained limited, public expectations of medicine were never high. This basic consensus achieved in the Middle Ages and codified in the *ars moriendi* survived down to the end of the nineteenth century, when secular trends and the burgeoning status of therapeutic medicine began to stimulate interest in mercy killing.

Thus, as the Middle Ages began to fade and the effects of the Renaissance started to be felt, a clear collective attitude toward suicide and euthanasia emerged. The medieval consensus was not without nuances. But the medieval mind, by conflating suicide, euthanasia, and the sixth commandment ("thou shalt not kill"), found it difficult to condone hastening a death, either by someone else's or one's own hands. By the onset of the sixteenth century, church, state, society, and medicine had forged an alliance that decisively rejected the taking of a life either by suicide or with medical assistance. This durable alliance would weather the Renaissance, the Reformation, and even the Enlightenment, lasting for the most part down to the early twentieth century. Only then would the venerable Christian consensus regarding a good death begin to unravel.

THE EARLY MODERN ERA

In the period between the fifteenth century and the end of the religious wars in the seventeenth century, Europe witnessed tremendous changes. The national monarchies of Spain, France, and England emerged as powerful political forces, while the temporal authority of the papacy steadily declined. Global exploration, technological innovation, scientific progress, economic expansion, and pioneering thought flourished. Included in the era's remarkable cultural ferment were debates over suicide in plays, poetry, novels, and philosophic treatises. At no prior time in history had suicide generated so much keen interest.

Yet, despite this widespread intellectual unrest, by the time of the eighteenth-century Enlightenment a major overhaul of Christian morality had not occurred. Suicide was never rehabilitated during this time span. Though the term "euthanasia" was used for the first time since classical antiquity, and the practice was discussed by luminaries such as Thomas More, suicide remained strictly forbidden and morally abhorrent.

In England alone, more than two hundred suicides appeared on the stage in a hundred plays between 1580 and 1620. A number of William Shakespeare's popular plays contained ruminations about the purpose of existence ("to be or not to be") as well as what might actually happen when human beings "shuffl'd off this mortal coil." Just before she kills herself, Cleopatra remarks: "Let's do it after the high Roman fashion," and Romeo and Juliet both dispatched themselves in the name of love. Writers such as Montaigne and Robert Burton treated suicide not as a matter of abstract morality but rather as a question of situational ethics. Did suicides always go to hell, as theologians preached? Was suicide due to diabolical possession, the disease of melancholy, or moral failure? "*Que sais-je?*" ("what do I know?") asked the sceptic Montaigne, admitting his inability to know positively if someone sinned by committing suicide. Was self-murder the same as killing, but under different circumstances? These thoughts were the first indications of a tendency that would blossom in the late nineteenth century, a secular movement to remove suicide from the domain of religion and redefine it as a topic of purely philosophic and medical concern.

The sixteenth and seventeenth centuries were revolutionary years in matters ranging from science to religion—yet the most fundamental ethical principles of Christianity stood unshaken, including the belief in the sanctity of life. This absence of radical change in conventional morality is particularly striking in view of the fact that these centuries were also a time of fierce religious dissent and conflict. Martin Luther's defiance of the Roman Catholic Church and the spread of the Protestant Reformation produced grave disagreements over issues of Christian doctrine, primarily questions related to how individuals merited God's grace and achieved salvation. Nonetheless, Protestant Reformers and Counter-Reformation Catholics overwhelmingly agreed with the medieval theory that suicide and euthanasia were such loathsome sins that only someone possessed by the devil or gripped by madness could commit these acts. Converting to Protestantism led pivotal figures such as Martin Luther, John Calvin, and Thomas Cranmer to jettison numerous Roman Catholic rituals and dogmas, but it did not cause them to defy the historic Catholic repudiation of suicide or euthanasia. If anything, Protestant theologians tended to be firmer in their opposition to suicide and euthanasia than Catholics. Believers in the unerring wisdom of scripture, Protestants saw no biblical justification for taking anyone's life to escape life's misfortunes. Catholic theologians, often impressed by the classical literature on suicide, were actually more willing to acknowledge that in certain circumstances an individual might reasonably want to die, such as virginal women who preferred death to dishonor.[11]

Science, too, led to rich intellectual ferment without causing any substantive upheaval in Christian morality. In the sixteenth and seventeenth centuries, scientific pioneers such as Copernicus, Kepler, Galileo, Harvey, and Newton often drew on the ideas of ancient philosophers in their efforts to transform the understanding of humanity's relationship to nature. In the process, the medieval cosmology based on the astronomy of Ptolemy and the physics of Aristotle increasingly came under attack, and it was finally replaced in the late seventeenth century by the Newtonian paradigm featuring a heliocentric universe governed by a universal, mathematical law of gravitational attraction.

However, just as their reformationist counterparts clung to traditional beliefs about the moral laws that regulated God's created world, so the leaders of the scientific revolution proved to be a distinctly unadventurous group when it came to questioning what rules of conduct ought to guide a Christian's life. Either they denounced the taking of one's life or (more commonly) were conspicuously silent on the subject.

THOMAS MORE

In the midst of these unsettling times, two well-known historical figures specifically raised the issue of euthanasia. The first was Thomas More (1478–1535), lord chancellor to King Henry VIII of England from 1529 to 1532. More was beheaded in 1535 for refusing to swear allegiance to Henry as the head of the Church of England. In *Utopia* (1515), his book about an ideal island realm, More described how the natives could take their own lives or ask others to do the deed if they were stricken by painful and incurable illnesses.

> If a disease is not only incurable but also distressing and agonizing without any cessation, then the priests and the public officials exhort the man, since he is now unequal to all life's duties, a burden to himself, and a trouble to others, and is living beyond the time of his death, to make up his mind not to foster the pest and plague any longer nor to hesitate to die now that life is torture to him but, relying on good hope, to free himself from this bitter life as from prison and the rack, or else voluntarily to permit others to free him. In this course he will act wisely since by death he will put an end not to enjoyment but to torture. . . . It will be a pious and holy action.

More's meaning seems clear: by taking their own lives to escape the physical torture of disease and disability, or allowing someone to administer poison, the residents of Utopia "lose nothing but suffering." So unambiguous do More's comments appear to be that several twentieth-century proponents of legalized euthanasia have cited More as a means of undercutting Catholic opposition to mercy killing.[12]

However, More's meaning in *Utopia* is not at all clear. His comments on euthanasia are amply overshadowed by the fact that More was a devout Roman Catholic who willingly died defending his church rather than go against papal authority. There is no evidence that he personally dissented from any church dogma. In 1534, when facing execution in the Tower of London, he utterly rejected suicide and even penned *A Dialogue of Comfort against Tribulation*, in which he dismissed all thoughts of suicide as due to temptation originating with the devil.

The nature of *Utopia* as a text is key to understanding More's superficial defense of euthanasia. There is so much that is fantastical in the book's contents that it is impossible to know what precisely More wanted his readers to take seriously or what More's own opinion of a particular matter was.

More himself was a difficult man to read: as a relative said about him, "few could see by his looke whether he spoke in earnest or in jeaste."[13] Only by arbitrarily lifting More's comments about euthanasia out of the book can the reader maintain that More favored euthanasia.

FRANCIS BACON

The influential scientist and philosopher Francis Bacon (1561–1626) also addressed the issue of euthanasia. Bacon, despite some equivocal remarks, did not endorse the practice of actively ending a patient's life. Bacon was the first in history since Roman historian Suetonius (c. 70–140 AD) in *The Lives of the Caesars* to use the term "euthanasia." Both Bacon and Suetonius employed the word in its etymological meaning, that is, to signify an easy death through the mitigation of pain rather than a death hastened by a physician through the administration of poison.[14]

At the same time, Bacon's criticism of the medical profession revealed how the art of medicine had changed since classical antiquity. To Bacon, the physicians of his day were guilty of not trying hard enough to find cures for diseases conventionally labeled as incurable. They were also prone, he complained, to "make a kind of scruple and religion to stay with the patient after he is given up," when they should have worked more assiduously "to mitigate the pains and torments of diseases . . . and when, all hope of recovery is gone, to help make a fair and easy passage from life." Bacon's remarks confirm that physicians in the early modern era, unlike their counterparts from antiquity, tended to stay with their patients until the bitter end. Yet, befitting a man whose disgust with the methods and theories of the professions of his time was legendary, Bacon faulted physicians for their lack of curiosity about ways of studying and defeating disease. His anti-medical comments also indicated that he wanted healers to be more concerned with the general welfare of the dying patient, what in the twentieth century would be called palliative care.

As the founder of the so-called scientific method in the natural sciences, Bacon thought his peers in medicine were little better than bumbling, uninquisitive quacks, and this colored his comments about them. Yet, unlike twentieth-century reformers who advocated euthanasia because they believed physicians did not do what was best for seriously ill patients, Bacon's low opinion of doctors did not transform him into an advocate of active mercy killing.

JOHN BUNYAN

As the seventeenth century wore on, the era's horrific religious wars gradually came to a close. So, too, the theological passions of the previous two centuries began to cool. In the wake of the often violent disagreements over Christian doctrine, the religious and legal prohibition against suicide remained unscathed. John Bunyan's *Pilgrim's Progress* (1678) was a landmark text that captured this consensus among European Christians. Bunyan's own life (1628–1688) was full of trials and tribulations. A preacher and soldier in the parliamentary army during the brutal English civil war, he was imprisoned twice (once for twelve years) and suffered severe bouts of both depression and physical illness. When he wrote in *Pilgrim's Progress* of its heroes being imprisoned in the "nasty and stinking" and "very dark dungeon" of Doubting Castle, and encouraged to commit suicide by "Giant Despair" to avoid torture and death, he could very well have been writing about his personal experiences. Bunyan concluded that placing one's faith in God enabled the Christian to combat the devil and forsake the superficial solution of suicide, even in the face of a painful and imminent death. These words proved to be powerful to countless Christians at a time when suicide seemed to be epidemic, particularly in Britain, which shortly would become known as the homeland of the melancholy that caused suicide.

The widespread popularity of Bunyan's views helps to account for the fate of poet John Donne's *Biathanatos* (1644), published posthumously. Donne (1572–1631) argued that examining suicide within the context of Christian theology revealed that "selfe-homicide" was not nearly as grave a sin as moralists thought, and might not even be a sin at all. To presume that someone who kills himself is damned is tantamount to reading the inscrutable mind of God, and therefore impossible. Donne also asked why society professed a faith in the sixth commandment's prohibition against murder when it simultaneously made exceptions for capital punishment and killing in wartime. Ultimately, however, *Biathanatos* fell far short of Donne's ordinary literary standards. It was read by few, and its subtleties were grasped by even fewer. Christians before and since Donne have found it supremely difficult to condone an act that seemed to say life was an individual's property, not God's. Suffering, whether of the physical or mental kind, was intended to be borne patiently rather than used as an excuse for exiting the world.

By the time the seventeenth century came to a close, a great deal of ink had been spilled over the question of suicide in the preceding two hundred years. Theologians, physicians, scientists, playwrights, poets, and novelists had analyzed its many dimensions. Most of the objections to the prohibition against suicide had to do with the severe punishments meted out to the bodies of suicides and their families. Disgust with these sanctions was steadily growing. Scepticism about society's institutions and customs was also mounting. Yet the cultural ferment of the early modern era had not fundamentally shaken belief in the Christian moral and ethical code. For the vast majority of European Christians, there was no sympathy for the handful of suicide apologists. Christian opponents of suicide believed that ownership of life resided in the Creator, and if human beings destroyed that life, they were committing a horrendous sin. It came down to the question: is one's life God's property, or is it one's own? Early modern Christians answered resoundingly that humans had mastery over what they did with their lives, except in regard to life itself.

The rest of the world tended to be as united as Christian Europeans in their opposition to suicide. Christendom's great foe, Islam, for example, threatened the very gates of Vienna in the sixteenth and seventeenth centuries, but Muslims utterly rejected the kind of reasoning Montaigne or John Donne indulged. Islam and the great religions of Asia found the notion that it was ethical to kill oneself to escape the sufferings of life incoherent. Within such cultural and intellectual contexts, there could be no possibility of approving either mercy killing or assisted suicide. As the eighteenth-century Enlightenment dawned, nothing could have been more alien to the mainstream Christian mentality than the modern-day conception of a right to die.

NOTES

1. Danielle Gourevitch, "Suicide among the Sick in Classical Antiquity," *Bulletin of the History of Medicine* 43 (1969): 501–518.

2. Edward J. Larson and Darrel W. Amundsen, *A Different Death: Euthanasia and the Christian Tradition* (Downers Grove, Ill.: InterVarsity Press, 1998), 31.

3. Ludwig Edelstein, "The Hippocratic Oath: Text, Translation, and Interpretation," in *Ancient Medicine: Selected Papers of Ludwig Edelstein*, ed. Owsei Temkin and C. Lilian Temkin (Baltimore: Johns Hopkins University Press, 1967), 23–53.

4. Roy Porter, *The Greatest Benefit to Mankind: A Medical History of Humanity* (New York: Norton, 1998), 62–63.

5. Larson and Amundsen, *A Different Death*, 54.

6. Gerald A. Larue, *Euthanasia and Religion: A Survey of the Attitudes of World Religions to the Right-to-Die* (Los Angeles: Hemlock Society, 1985), 137.

7. Georges Minois, *History of Suicide: Voluntary Death in Western Culture*, trans. Lydia G. Cochrane (Baltimore: Johns Hopkins University Press, 1999), 9.

8. Porter, *The Greatest Benefit to Mankind*, 112–113.

9. Pat Jalland, *Death in the Victorian Family* (New York: Oxford University Press, 1996), 18.

10. Jalland, *Death in the Victorian Family*, 18.

11. Minois, *History of Suicide*, 122–127.

12. Thomas More, "Utopia," in *The Right to Die Debate: A Documentary History*, ed. Marjorie B. Zucker (Westport, Conn.: Greenwood Press, 1999), 228.

13. Peter Ackroyd, *The Life of Thomas More* (New York: Doubleday, 1998), 177.

14. Robert P. Hudson, "The Many Faces of Euthanasia," *Medical Heritage* 2 (1986): 102–107.

2

THIS TROUBLESOME SHORE

The almost unanimous cultural disapproval of suicide and euthanasia may have remained fairly steady between the Renaissance and the eighteenth-century Enlightenment, but it began to fray around the edges in the 1700s. In the eighteenth century, suicide became one of the most fiercely debated topics among Western intellectuals.[1] Between the end of the wars of Louis XIV in 1715 and the outbreak of the French Revolution in 1789, leading thinkers such as Voltaire, Montesquieu, d'Alembert, and Hume either justified voluntary death or in the very least attacked the legal punishments for suicide as barbaric, unjust, and useless. For the first time since classical antiquity, secular, naturalist, individualist, and anti-clerical rationalizations for euthanasia were voiced by more than a tiny handful of prominent people.

By the end of the eighteenth century, this readiness to endorse suicide as an affirmation of individual autonomy and a rationalist protest against conventional morality as defined by the leading churches was still a minority position. Nonetheless, a milestone had been reached in the history of Western attitudes toward death and dying. The ancient Greek and Roman belief that suicide was a triumphant victory over human nature and a legitimate exercise of individual rights enjoyed a significant revival. Suicide's popularity waxed and waned over the next three hundred years, but it would never disappear entirely, and it would help to create the conditions responsible for the spectacular rise in support for euthanasia in the twentieth century.

THE "ENGLISH MALADY"

In the face of overwhelming condemnation from theologians of virtually all Christian denominations, more and more Europeans expressed permissive opinions about suicide in the early eighteenth century. The word "suicide" had been coined in 1642 by the English doctor and author Thomas Browne (1605–1682). Browne depicted the suicides of noteworthy pagan Romans and Greeks as noble and rational, and thus as fundamentally different from the sinful and abhorrent acts of "self-killing" that evidently occurred every day. The neologism "suicide" was used intermittently in England for the balance of the seventeenth century. In 1734, the term first appeared in French. When it did, it signaled the origins of the perception that murdering someone and the taking of one's life were not identical from a moral standpoint. The notion that voluntary death no longer deserved grave religious, legal, and social condemnation started to take root in the eighteenth century, naturally stimulating discussion about the many varied motives behind suicide and the means the civil law adopted to discourage people from killing themselves.

Much of the discussion of suicide was due to the perception that it was epidemic throughout the British Isles. As one Englishman in 1702 noted gloomily in his diary, " 'Tis . . . sad to Consider how many of this Nation have murdered themselves of late." In an age before modern statistical methods, it was easy for people to form the impression that England was the land of suicide. Even before the British physician George Cheyne wrote his 1733 book of the same name, the theory of the "English Malady" had been widely accepted. Cheyne's thesis was that the English people, inhabiting an island with poor weather, were naturally melancholy. Their morose temperament, when combined with the growing secularism of the age, led them to kill themselves in disproportionate numbers. Cheyne's ideas clearly touched a nerve among literate Europeans of his day. A Frenchman who arrived in London in 1727 and found the weather depressing confessed that, if he had been born an Englishman, he would have already committed suicide. Cheyne's thesis that geographic and climatic factors determine character and personality mirrored the development of the social sciences: the attempt to use science to explain social conditions. His views also reflected the dawning eighteenth-century theory that human feelings were deeply affected by natural causes. This theory would be used throughout the eighteenth century to undermine the religious interpretation of suicide as a heinous sin and an affront to God's gift of life.[2]

Interest in suicide in the early eighteenth century reached unprecedented levels, thanks in large part to the rise of the popular press. As cities such as London grew rapidly in population, the number of newspapers multiplied. Some papers published as many as 15,000 copies per issue. Europe's first successful daily appeared in London in 1702, and by 1792 there were sixteen dailies in the city. By 1750, the annual sale of newspapers in England was 7.3 million. Rome, Moscow, Paris, Copenhagen, and the American colonies followed London's example as the century wore on. Even Germany, provincial by comparison, had 126 newspapers in 1775. Suicides were recorded in the bills of mortality, which in turn were published in the burgeoning press. Popular interest tended to focus on the suicides of the rich and powerful. It was common knowledge that the poor, sick, and disabled, mired in misery, often took their own lives. But when members of the advantaged classes with relatively fewer reasons to end their own lives killed themselves, it naturally fostered the belief that suicide was a mounting social problem and was often an involuntary reaction to factors beyond the individual's control.

The impact of the press on suicide had another, more long-lasting effect. Press coverage of suicide introduced the public to the human-interest story, which made suicide seem more mundane than before. Those who committed suicide also looked less like criminals and more like victims, people who could not help themselves. Newspapers repeatedly reported cases of suicide due to the timeless yet quotidian situations of marital unhappiness, unrequited love, family quarrels, painful sickness, financial reverses, and the like. The value-neutral tone in which these stories were reported generally discouraged readers from passing moral judgments. The effect was less approval of suicide than acceptance of it as a fact of human existence and, for some, a belief that religious definitions of suicide were oversimplistic. This nonjudgmental characteristic of the popular press has continued down to the present day, when media accounts of heartrending cases of suffering individuals are journalistic staples.

In the late seventeenth and early eighteenth centuries, however, growing press reports of suicide convinced many that atheism was spreading. "Religion is so dead," exclaimed the Princess Palatine in 1699, "that all the young men desire to be considered atheists." Continental Europe was being ravaged by the scourge of suicide, she lamented, and she had no doubt it was due to an upsurge in godlessness.[3] The princess, like so many of her educated contemporaries, felt deluged by stories of suicide printed in newspapers. She was not alone in linking changing attitudes toward suicide to the faltering credibility of organized religion among literate, early eighteenth-century Europeans. As for the upsurge in godlessness that the princess felt called to remark upon, an Anglican bishop wrote in the early eighteenth century: "there never was an age since the death of Christ, never once since the commencement of this history of the world, in which atheism and infidelity have been more generally confessed."[4]

THE ENLIGHTENMENT

The corrosion of belief in accepted religious values regarding suicide was readily encouraged by many philosophers of the eighteenth-century Enlightenment who were dissatisfied with the religious, political, and social status quo. These individuals influenced the way many thinkers in later centuries interpreted key social issues. Enlightenment theorists tended to admire science as a method for developing new technologies that would increase human happiness, health, and prosperity. Trying to reform conditions on earth by improving the quality of life for society's unfortunates was a goal most people of common sense supported, but it led many Enlightenment figures to emphasize living in the world at the expense of concern for the hereafter. In the words of medical historian Erwin Ackerknecht, death to an Enlightenment thinker "was a very different and far more frightening thing than it had been for his ancestors. To them it was primarily a portal to a better world." For admirers of Enlightenment ideas, death instead was "a kind of secularized hell," a natural process that scientific medicine, it was hoped, would find ways of making less fearsome.[5]

Enlightenment philosophers also respected science because they believed it was a more reliable means for determining truth than theological speculation. For example, in his 1733 *Letters on England*, Voltaire (1694–1778) repeatedly compared the scientific method based on experimentation and inductive reasoning with what he believed were the sterile debates of theologians (almost always Roman Catholic) about such things as the nature of the soul or the doctrine of transubstantiation, which held that the sacramental elements of bread and wine were transformed into the body and blood of Christ during the Mass. He insisted that, if only human beings followed the rules for determining scientific knowledge instead of quarreling over religious issues, war itself could be averted. Organized religion, according to Voltaire, was the chief source of conflict and main impediment to peace, truth, and justice.

Science and the expanding body of knowledge about the universe gathered by explorers and travelers also bred a kind of cultural relativism most manifest in Montesquieu's *Persian Letters* (1721) or Denis Diderot's *Supplement to the Voyage of Bougainville* (1772). As people became increasingly educated about parts of the world never before discovered by Europeans, they became less inclined to believe that the value systems and institutions of their own Christian civilization were unique and beyond questioning.

Montesquieu (1689–1755) was an eminent example of someone who used cultural relativism to launch a frontal attack on conventional attitudes toward suicide. A brilliant satirist of French social and political institutions, he dismissed the idea that someone who commits suicide harmed society or hindered God's providential plan, and he invoked what later would be called an appeal to personal autonomy. "If I am laden with sorrow, misery, and contempt," Montesquieu wondered, what possible purpose could be served by depriving him of a "remedy which lies in my hands?" Or, as his countryman Voltaire put it, "the Republic will do without me as it did before I was born."[6]

To Voltaire, Montesquieu, and others of the Enlightenment, suicide was chiefly a question of individual liberty. They were optimistic that individuals, with the proper education, could make rational choices, even if the decisions concerned ending one's own life. Voltaire applied this reasoning to cases of suicide for elderly people suffering from "intolerable pain," cases highly similar to those frequently cited in modern debates over euthanasia. In doing so, he also indicated how killing oneself as an exercise in individual liberty could easily become confused with ending lives that were no longer useful to society. What was the point, he argued, in extending the lives of old people by operating on them, when in their dotage they continued "to dribble, and shuffle along for [another] year, a burden to [themselves] and others"?

No one defended suicide as a personal right more strongly than Voltaire's contemporary David Hume (1711–1776), the Scottish philosopher. Due to Hume's own reluctance to face the fierce opposition he expected his pro-suicide argument would spark, his *Essays on Suicide* were not published in France until 1770 and in England until 1777, a year after his death. His fears were well-grounded, as his tract unleashed a torrent of invective and denunciation from numerous religious figures across the denominational spectrum. The strident reaction to Hume's defense of suicide signaled that, as the eighteenth century drew to a close, secularist Enlightenment philosophy was increasingly under attack.

Suicide was beyond criticism, Hume contended, because, in the natural scheme of things, all voluntary deaths were the result of the laws that governed the universe. Suicide provided individuals with their "chance for happiness in life" and freed them from "all danger of misery." Anticipating twentieth-century justifications of assisted suicide, Hume added that the Mosaic commandment against killing never referred to suicide, only the taking of another's life.

In Hume's thinking about suicide, the decision to kill oneself did not serve solely personal purposes. As he wrote: "Suppose that it is no longer in my power to promote the interest of society, suppose that I am a burden to it, suppose that my life hinders some person from being much more useful to society. In such cases, my resignation of life must not only be innocent, but laudable."[7] Life could easily become a "burden" because of age, sickness, and misfortune, and when it did, "annihilation" was preferable. To Hume, suicide may have been a remedy for the ills of life, but in his discussion of the issue, the boundaries between a right to suicide and a social duty to kill oneself were never terribly clear.

Enlightenment philosophers not only justified suicide as socially desirable and a matter of personal choice, but they also explained it by citing the theory that material factors caused a person to commit suicide. Based on his belief that geography heavily shaped human nature, Montesquieu contended that the English malady of suicide was due to physiological causes, what he called "a distemper, being connected with the physical state of the [bodily] machine. . . . In all probability it is a defect of the filtration of the nervous juice."[8]

Montesquieu's Enlightenment colleague Baron d'Holbach (1723–1789) took the materialist argument even further. He relentlessly opposed the religious theory that suicide was an act against nature. The decision to commit suicide was due to "a temperament soured by chagrin, a bilious constitution, a melancholy habit, a defect in the organization, a derangement in the whole machine." Moral teachings are useless in the face of these tendencies, he contended. In words that applied to later rationalizations of euthanasia, d'Holbach wrote: "if the same power that obliges all intelligent beings to cherish their existence, renders that of man so painful and so cruel that he finds it insupportable, he quits his species; order is destroyed for him, and he accomplishes a decree of nature that wills he should no longer exist."[9]

The theory that suicide is determined by biological or physiological factors and thus was a purely natural act convinced many eighteenth-century thinkers that the laws governing suicide were unjust. When judges ordered the bodies of suicides to be hauled through the streets and their property confiscated, weren't they incongruously "punishing the effects of madness," Montesquieu asked. The opinions of such people as Montesquieu coincided with the ways the popular press sympathetically reported tales of suicide. The result by the early 1700s was that judges were increasingly softening their decisions regarding the reasons behind suicides. In many localities, judges ruled that those who killed themselves were not guilty by reason of insanity. This pattern in legal judgments reflected the mounting tendency to ascribe voluntary death to natural causes rather than the influence of Satan.

It also reflected a diffuse distaste with the penalties courts imposed on not just the bodies of the deceased, but the property of the suicide's family. Many Europeans, including at least one monarch, had concluded by the eighteenth century that the laws governing suicide were exceedingly harsh and ineffective. In 1751, Frederick the Great of Prussia, admirer of Voltaire and other Enlightenment thinkers, annulled the customary punishments for suicide. Even those who were less willing to question the moral prohibitions against suicide thought these laws were barbaric and had outlived any useful purpose.

The view that the laws governing suicide were inhumane and useless received its most eloquent expression in the works of the Italian criminologist Cesare Beccaria (1738–1794). The political liberty of human beings, according to Beccaria, demanded that punishment be tailored to the individual, fit the crime, and serve to deter others from doing the same thing. In 1764, his highly influential *On Crimes and Punishments* was published in Italian. Beccaria reasoned that punishing the suicide's body by dragging it through the streets or driving a stake through the cadaver's heart was as ridiculous as whipping a statue. Similarly, confiscating the property of the deceased was merely punishing the innocent. For Beccaria, the body of law concerning suicide throughout Western civilization failed miserably on all three counts and deserved to be abolished.

These Enlightenment beliefs about the laws against suicide tended to reinforce an emerging anti-clerical spirit that was perhaps most evident in prerevolutionary France. Despite what the Princess Palatine and others might have thought, this form of anti-clericalism was less a derivative of atheism than a generalized scepticism toward traditional Christian teaching about how to live a moral and ethical life. At its roots, anti-clericalism was often an assertion of individual rights in the face of church teachings that stressed obedience to religious doctrine. The outcome was a sharp controversy that lasted for much of the eighteenth century. Some Enlightenment thinkers openly defended an individual's right to suicide. Others merely expressed sympathy for those unfortunates who turned to voluntary death because they were plunged in acute despair, or for the families of suicides who had their property confiscated. Ranged against them was a host of theologians who sometimes took a nuanced approach to suicide, but who ultimately defended the orthodox position that suicide was a crime against both God and the state.

The legacy of Enlightenment-era writings on suicide was undeniably powerful, exerting an influence down to the present day. The most immediate impact of Enlightenment writing on suicide was the repeal or mitigation of the common-law punishments against suicide. In post-revolutionary America, suicide was in fact decriminalized, a reflection of popular unhappiness with the severity of anti-suicide laws. None of this could have been possible without the Enlightenment defense of individual freedom of thought, a luminous example of the human spirit's refusal to succumb to censorship and other types of political and clerical intimidation.

However, as historian Lester Crocker has noted, "on the question of suicide, as in other matters, the Enlightenment was unable to achieve true unity of thought."[10] When all the strands of the Enlightenment's intellectual legacy were woven into the theories of a single person (such as Montesquieu), the result was far from consistent. Materialists such as d'Holbach sought mightily to make suicide a subject of scientific inquiry rather than theological analysis. They attempted to normalize suicide as an act that stemmed from purely natural causes. On the other hand, they also defended the autonomy of individuals to commit suicide. They argued that taking one's life was an eminently rational act under many circumstances and therefore was immune to religious condemnation. In terms of assisted suicide, if individuals were afflicted with the pains and sufferings of old age, why were they prohibited from asking someone to help them kill themselves?

Yet, if the decision to commit suicide (or ask to be put out of one's misery) is governed by blind natural law, how can it then be a free choice? How could such a decision be simultaneously the product of individual reason and determined by mechanical natural forces? How, in other words, could human beings be at one and the same time both an exception to and governed by natural laws? In their haste to erase the distinction between human beings and the laws of nature, Enlightenment philosophers undermined their own appeals to moral freedom as the chief quality that separated them from the rest of nature.

In the end analysis, the Enlightenment thinkers' passionate defiance of tyranny and their backing of individual rights (especially in the case of suicide) have resonated down to the present day, but they were merely mortal when it came to erecting new theories that made coherent, systematic sense of the world. Nor were these contradictions unique to the eighteenth century. They would resurface during the nineteenth and twentieth centuries in the thought of euthanasia advocates who similarly used the newest trends in science (such as Darwinian evolutionary theory) as weapons in their struggles against long-standing religious taboos.

ROMANTICISM

As the eighteenth century came to a close, there were signs that public patience with Enlightenment dissent was wearing thin. Many concluded that the French Revolution in 1789, the Reign of Terror (1793–1794), and the militaristic horrors of the Napoleonic wars (1799–1815) could be traced to Enlightenment ideas, unleashing a reaction against what was popularly believed to be the eighteenth-century overemphasis on reason and intellect. This reaction, often called Romanticism, was no more unified than Enlightenment thought, yet most Romantics shared the conviction that Enlightenment reason without feeling and faith was an arid human faculty. In 1823, the German writer Johann Wolfgang von Goethe (1749–1832) went so far as to praise superstition as "the poetry of life. . . . Superstition does no harm to the poet, because he can turn his half-delusions to advantage in a variety of ways." Thanks to views such as Goethe's, religion enjoyed a revival of sorts. Some Romantics turned to Catholicism, some to Protestantism, some to medieval art and culture, and some to Oriental exoticism.

In a sign of the times, the Vicomte René de Chateaubriand (1768–1848) published his 1802 masterpiece *The Genius of Christianity*, a best-seller that attributed singular artistic greatness and spiritual truth to the church. Its subtitle summed up its thesis: "the poetic and moral beauties of the Christian religion." The Romantics' belief systems were rarely as orthodox as Chateaubriand's, but they were normally imbued with a respect for the religious instinct in human beings, something they felt had been unfairly denigrated by secular Enlightenment philosophy.

The popularity of *The Genius of Christianity* was enhanced by Napoleon Bonaparte's having made the Roman Catholic Church once again the established church in France in 1801. Yet the power of Chateaubriand's book to convert people to Christianity persisted long after the Romantic era ended.[11]

JOHN WESLEY

No individual was more responsible for paving the way for a spiritual reawakening than English theologian John Wesley (1703–1791). Wesley introduced Christians to Methodism, and in the process profoundly affected the lives of millions on both sides of the Atlantic Ocean. Methodism spread rapidly after 1739 in England and North America, formally separating from the Church of England in 1791. Wesley is believed to have preached over 40,000 sermons, some to audiences as large as 20,000. His message defied Enlightenment rationalism. Wesley also challenged eighteenth-century scepticism about core religious teachings and the Enlightenment theory that people were essentially good but just misled and uneducated. Human nature was instead depraved, Wesley maintained. The good news he preached was that human nature could be redeemed through the abandonment of all pride. Faith in the sacrifice of Jesus Christ was key for Wesley. He taught passionately that religion should be "plain, artless, simple! Meekness, temperance, patience, faith, and love—be these my highest gifts."[12]

Little wonder that Wesley vigorously attacked Hume's position on suicide and endorsed the Christian condemnation of suicide as self-murder. Suicide, as he saw it, was the worst kind of pride and selfishness. Other Christian churches were not always happy with Wesley's teaching, however. Anglicans accused him and his followers of inadvertently causing suicidal melancholy because of their heavy emphasis on hell and eternal damnation. Wesley's Methodists fervently supported the orthodox Christian position that the devil was ultimately responsible for cases of self-murder and could only be defeated through ardent faith in Christ. As one Methodist confessed in 1763, Satan tempted him to use his razor on himself one day, "but something within answered. No murderer hath eternal life abiding in him. . . . At length I threw the razor on the ground, and fell on my knees. God soon heard me, and rebuked the destroyer."[13]

Wesley's colleague George Whitefield (1714–1770), who carried Methodism to the thirteen British colonies of North America, ensured that Wesley's prohibition of suicide became a cardinal article of Christian faith there. Between the 1730s and 1760s, ideas similar to Wesley's fanned the fires of evangelical Christianity first fueled by the Massachusetts preacher Jonathan Edwards. This chapter in American history, often called the First Great Awakening, was characterized by the religious teaching that surrendering to God's will led eventually to an intense emotional conversion experience. Unlike in Europe, evangelicalism in America helped to foster political reform. New colleges were founded, including the College of New Jersey (now Princeton University) and the College of Rhode Island (now Brown University). Religious dissent encouraged many to question orthodoxy in politics and forms of social organization. The participation of women and African Americans in religious activities became increasingly acceptable. Later, in the nineteenth century, evangelicalism inspired many Americans (especially women's reform groups) to attack prostitution, slavery, and the abuse of alcohol. In the meantime, the command to submit to

God's will was readily accepted by countless American colonists and undermined eighteenth-century rationales for suicide, even as many of the newly created American states ended criminal penalties for suicide.

Methodism and other examples of Christian revivalism in the late eighteenth century indicated that the early confidence of Enlightenment secularism rested on shaky ground. "Just now," Voltaire wrote in 1733, "people are so indifferent to [theological disputes] that there is not much chance of success for a new religion or a revived one." Wesleyism and the waves of religious awakening in America that continued well into the nineteenth century proved that Voltaire was better at composing verse and satire than predicting the future of religion.

Assaults on Enlightenment theories of suicide gathered powerful momentum by the turn of the nineteenth century. Some attacks came from secular quarters. The German philosopher Immanuel Kant (1724–1804) argued that morality was based on two chief principles: first, that human beings should be treated as ends in themselves and never as means to an end, and second, that a moral act is something that must serve as the basis for a universal law. Suicide failed both tests, according to Kant, and thus was immoral. Morality trumped any self-interest when it came to dying. Any form of suicide (such as physician-assisted suicide) violated universal morality, knowledge of which, Kant argued, resided in each human being's heart and mind.

MADAME DE STAËL

The backlash against eighteenth-century permissiveness toward suicide is equally evident in the writings of Madame de Staël (1766–1817), the gifted daughter of French royal minister Jacques Necker. Madame de Staël was influenced by the growing romantic mood of late eighteenth-century Europe, most popularly expressed in Goethe's novel *The Sorrows of Young Werther* (1774). *Werther* was the story of a young man's suicide when he refused to live without the married woman he passionately loved. Like many of her age, de Staël admired the idea of suicide for love and in 1796 defended the act as noble and courageous. However, by 1813 she had largely changed her mind. No longer did she believe that there was something exquisitely sensitive and stirringly philosophical about killing oneself over love. She argued instead that people who commit suicide were neither noble nor worthy of condemnation; rather, suicides were to be pitied.

Undoubtedly, taking one's own life meant one was not afraid of death, but people who stoically accepted their suffering were generally stronger and more admirable individuals. In words that applied as much to voluntary euthanasia as they did to suicide, de Staël noted that physical suffering did not lead most often to a desire to kill oneself, but rather a willingness to face suffering and all its torments if fellow human beings provided care and comfort. Suffering, she concluded, was inevitable, and ought to be welcomed as beneficial. It provided the opportunity to "consecrate oneself to one's fellow creatures," whereas suicide was little else than a selfish, anti-social act.

In her later writings, de Staël neatly summarized the anti-Enlightenment consensus about suicide that had crystallized by the early nineteenth century in educated circles: few wanted to return to the medieval punishments for killing oneself, and many believed suicides were indeed more to be pitied than vilified, but few remained sympathetic to Enlightenment justifications of taking one's own life to escape the physical and emotional pain of disability, disease, or impending death. The religious attitude toward suicide and euthanasia remained intact, despite the efforts of secularist eighteenth-century thinkers to normalize these acts. Dying continued to be seen as a test of courage and religious virtue. And euthanasia was still mainly understood to refer to a "good death" for Christians anxious to die in a state of grace.

Despite the heated debates over suicide throughout the eighteenth century, nothing had fundamentally altered the fact that for centuries Christians feared hell more than death. What worried Christians most as death approached were not the bodily "stings of death" but the prospect of dying "alienated from the Life of God," as the Puritan minister Cotton Mather wrote in 1723. Some forms of Christianity, such as New England Puritanism, by incessantly stressing human depravity and the finality of divine justice, did less than other churches in allaying fears of what might happen when people were "loosed from this troublesome Shore." But even Puritans, afraid of the terrors of hell that potentially awaited them, were more worried about what lay on the other side of death than they were about the pain and discomfort accompanying the physical process of dying. Until that changed, public opinion would never approve of assisted suicide, much less mercy killing.

All in all, then, as the nineteenth century began to unfold, Christian optimism remained the "principal weapon against the fear of death."[14] Conventional Christian attitudes toward death had successfully weathered the storm of Enlightenment criticism. Euthanasia continued to signify either the art of dying well in the face of divine judgment or the efforts of physicians to make the terminal stage of life more comfortable without hastening the process. The basic meaning of euthanasia dating back to the inception of the Christian era held fast.

VICTORIAN EVANGELISM

By the early Victorian era, most Christians still viewed suicide as a sin against God. Mercy killing was thought to be an even more heinous crime. If anything, in the nineteenth century these sentiments grew stronger throughout the Anglo-American world and beyond, due to the influence of the Christian Evangelical movement. Evangelical values of sobriety, discipline, duty, and individual accountability had a powerful effect on mores in Europe and America, deeply affecting society at large. Under these circumstances, the possibility of challenges to orthodox opinions about euthanasia was exceedingly remote, despite revolutionary developments in medical theory and practice.

The Evangelical spirit that accompanied the rise of Methodism in the eighteenth century enjoyed widespread acceptance in the nineteenth century on both sides of the Atlantic Ocean. In the United States, the Second Great Awakening swept the nation in the early nineteenth century, peaking in the 1830s. Starting at a revivalist meeting in Kentucky in 1801, the movement featured Methodist and Baptist preachers who taught that everyone was responsible for one's own soul and nobody was beyond redemption, no matter how sinful. Preachers also taught the virtues of sobriety, piety, and hard work, but above all they predicted that Christ's coming was at hand and that Christians should prepare themselves for the event. Conversions multiplied over the years. In 1784, there were 14,000 Methodists. By 1844, there were more than a million. Eastern establishment ministers took a dim view of the emotionalism of the Second Great Awakening, but they shared with the Evangelicals a militant commitment to social reform based on the moral message that virtue must be made to triumph throughout the nation. The reformist fervor of the Second Great Awakening spawned the abolitionist campaign against the institution of slavery. It also inspired men and women to swear off alcohol. At its peak a decade after its founding in 1826, the Evangelical American Temperance Society numbered 8,000 auxiliaries and 1.5 million members, one out of every ten Americans.[15]

Evangelicalism shaped the model of a "good death" for countless Christians. The Evangelical approach to death was a throwback to the Catholic *ars moriendi* tradition of the Middle Ages, but it also revitalized that tradition with a renewed piety and emotionalism. Evangelicals believed that humans ordinarily were mired in sin, but Christ's sacrifice on the cross had atoned for human sins and taught Christians that salvation lay in conversion to Christ's message through prayer, repentance, and diligent Bible study. Patient, stoical resignation to the suffering in death was often perceived as a sign that God had shed his grace on the dying individual. Thus, death could be the most significant moment in a person's life, a providential opportunity to convert at the last minute and achieve everlasting salvation. The Evangelical emphasis on sin, judgment, and the torments of hell overshadowed the painful ordeals that many endured when dying in the nineteenth century, stifling the temptation of those around the bedside to put the dying person out of his or her misery. An Evangelical death, in other words, could be a "triumphant death." Death held few terrors for the Evangelical.[16]

This Evangelical interpretation of a good death was deeply internalized by many nineteenth-century Christians. Victorian-era Christians believed fervently that a good death should take place at home, so family members and friends could say their farewells. They also believed a good death meant there had been sufficient time to tie up earthly matters. In a good death, the person remained lucid and conscious enough to beg forgiveness for sins and display the strength of character in suffering that would inspire others to follow his or her example.

This model of the good death proved remarkably tenacious even in the face of dreadfully unhappy deaths, such as the 1850 demise of four-year-old Jessy Gladstone, daughter of British Prime Minister William Gladstone. Jessy Gladstone died of tubercular meningitis and, in her last months of life, suffered terribly from pain, fever, and severe convulsions. Her final six hours of life were harrowing as fierce convulsions repeatedly gripped her small body, culminating just before she died in one prolonged convulsion for thirty minutes. All the while, Jessy's parents, family, and attending physician frantically did what they could to ease her pain, but even their doctor ultimately resorted to literally praying that "the passage of the departing spirit should be quickened."

William Gladstone struggled mightily to reconcile his deep Christian faith with the personal tragedy of Jessy's death. He found it extremely difficult to imagine that the death of this much-loved and blameless child served some divine purpose. But in the end, though grief-stricken, he concluded that it was God's "especial pleasure to remove her" to a place where earthly sorrows no longer existed. Jessy's death fell far short of the ideal Christian good death, but it was still considered a stroke of providence, the true meaning of which escaped human understanding. Resignation to God's will, and the consoling thought of being reunited someday, prevailed over the temptation to cut short her suffering by hastening her death.[17]

Evangelical teaching about the unfathomable meaning of suffering in death was echoed in nineteenth-century Catholic theology. Catholicism flourished after mid-century reports of miracle healings and sightings of the

Virgin Mary. The Jesus whom most Catholics of the mid-nineteenth century were taught to worship was the suffering Jesus. In sermon after sermon, priests told their parishioners to "meditate upon your suffering Jesus." One Boston priest told his audience: "God can give us no greater proof of His love than by sending afflictions."[18] "Joy born of affliction" was the attitude Christians were supposed to adopt when sick or dying. But joy was exceedingly difficult to feel when one was faced with horrible and heart-wrenching spectacles such as Jessy Gladstone's death.

DEATH, DISEASE, AND MEDICINE
IN THE NINETEENTH CENTURY

In the Victorian era, as in earlier periods in history, death was an ever-present reality, ready to strike anyone at any moment. "In life we are in the midst of death," wrote a Maine farmer in 1859. Nineteenth-century society was wracked by a wide variety of deadly diseases and infirmities that bewilderingly struck at young and old, male and female, rich and poor alike. This doleful reality was exacerbated by the fact that, during epidemics, the rate of mortality often spiked suddenly, spreading fear and sadness everywhere. In 1858, a New York State schoolteacher noted: "the grim messenger has been at work all over the land calling for his thousands. The lovely child has been taken from its sports; the youth has been taken from its circle of loved ones; the teacher from his arduous duties; the lawyer from the bar, the doctor from his office, the statesman from the senate chamber."[19]

Even when epidemics subsided, death steadily stalked the land. Antisepsis, the prevention of infection in wounds, was introduced in the 1880s. Until then, people died in droves from the spread of bacteria, especially in wartime. Over 100,000 Union soldiers are estimated to have perished from wounds during the U.S. Civil War.[20] In England, puerperal fever (infection acquired during birthing) took the lives of about five mothers for every thousand children born alive. Tuberculosis, a chronic, painful, and debilitating disease, killed more people than smallpox and cholera combined for much of the nineteenth century. Some writers romanticized deaths due to tuberculosis, but the stark suffering and drawn-out deaths of tuberculosis patients were anything but poetic. Though pneumonia (the "old man's friend") often intervened to cut short the agony of dying patients in the pre-antibiotic era, countless people still died "hard deaths" in the nineteenth century. Child mortality rates were much higher in the nineteenth century than today, and in the face of such baffling suffering, one might expect that enthusiasm for legal euthanasia would have been at an all-time peak. But it was not, and the reason was the cultural climate of the time. The Victorian era's religious precepts shaped the approach of people such as the Gladstone family to the admittedly harrowing and seemingly meaningless deaths of desperately loved ones.

Thus, nineteenth-century men and women tended to find meaning in death in religiously informed routines and ideals that defined it as an escape from the world's sadness, an inscrutable decision of providence that demanded human resignation. Death was thought of as the end to a spiritual pilgrimage filled with the "trembling hope" of heaven, no matter how frightening the prospect of hell. The Evangelical theory that death was to be accepted rather than lamented was reinforced even when witnesses to death described it in nonreligious terms. To many humble and marginally literate people in the nineteenth century, death meant a release from temporal misery as much as it represented a stepping stone on the way to heaven. "All she wanted was ease," a neighbor remarked about an Alabama woman who died in 1854.[21] If there was a lesson to the presence of death and the prevalence of terminal diseases in the nineteenth century, it was that the average person could never be prepared enough when this fateful moment struck.

One major reason that religious interpretations of dying reigned supreme was the pervasive realization that licensed physicians could do little for their seriously ill patients other than mitigate their pain with opium or other narcotics. The great breakthrough for medicine did not occur until the 1930s and 1940s, when antibiotics were discovered. Before the twentieth century, the only genuinely effective therapies physicians had at their disposal were quinine for malaria, digitalis for dropsy, lime juice for scurvy, and vaccination for smallpox. The medical profession was virtually helpless when it came to patients suffering from the killer diseases of the nineteenth century: syphilis, cholera, tuberculosis, pneumonia, diphtheria, to say nothing of cancer, diabetes, and cerebrovascular diseases. Mortality rates from many infectious conditions began to decline in the late nineteenth century, but that was due more to improvements in diet, sanitation, and preventive hygiene than curative medicine. By then, doctors had learned a great deal about how to prevent diseases from occurring in the first place, and their clinical skills at diagnosing different illnesses were sharply improving. But when faced with individual patients in agony and in danger of dying, they were essentially powerless. In Jessy Gladstone's case, her physician administered an opium-laced patent medicine, which briefly eased her pain, and calomel, which was supposed to ease her constipation. Still, except for an ability to diagnose the illness and predict its eventual course, nineteenth-century doctors were plainly ill-equipped to ward off death.

This state of therapeutic ineffectiveness had existed since time immemorial, but its impact was particularly glaring in the Victorian era because, on so many other fronts, organized medicine was making impressive strides. In the nineteenth century, physicians began forming occupational organizations, establishing educational standards for medical schools, founding professional journals, and driving alternative health-care competitors out of business. At the same time, brilliant pioneer doctors discovered cutting-edge methods of diagnosis, prognosis, and experimental medicine. This medical revolution had started in Paris after the 1789 revolution. There, physicians such as Philippe Pinel, René Laennec, Claude Bernard, and Louis Pasteur overthrew centuries-old theories of health care and introduced the first recognizably modern ideas about disease. Important new devices such as the stethoscope, ophthalmoscope, and X-ray were invented. Surgery benefited immeasurably from the introduction of anesthesia and antisepsis. The laboratory suddenly became an important site for determining what caused illness. Likewise, the hospital ceased being a place where poor people came to die and emerged as an institution that symbolized the felicitous combination of science, compassion, and care. By the end of the nineteenth century, the center for scientific medicine had shifted from France to Germany, but the profession's march of progress continued into the twentieth century. Doctors knew more than ever before what caused disease and disability. This remarkable progress, however, stood in stark contrast to organized medicine's inability to save lives, a situation that had not changed much throughout history.

NINETEENTH-CENTURY EUTHANASIA

The state of medicine in the nineteenth century left physicians in an anomalous position. On the one hand, the public viewed doctors as unprecedentedly knowledgeable, and this made them frequent visitors to a patient's bedside. On the other hand, doctors time and again had to share the deathbed scene with clergy and other interested parties. But it would be a mistake to characterize the relationship between doctors and clients as inherently antagonistic. Throughout the nineteenth and well into the twentieth century, a moral and ethical consensus tended to unite physicians and public, whether the topic was euthanasia, birth control, or any other contentious social issue. Many nineteenth-century physicians were devout

Christians who recognized that a patient's strong faith could help to "disarm death of its terrors."[22] Historically, some members of the medical profession have played instrumental roles in the social reform movements of the last two centuries, including the euthanasia and birth control movements, but until recently the vast majority of physicians have shared the socially conservative values of the public they served.

What physicians could offer was concern for the patient's overall well-being and personal life. This psychological dimension to the doctor-patient relationship has a therapeutic power that is now well-documented. Physicians could function as a friend of the family and a source of indispensable moral support. They could also ensure that the bedroom was well ventilated and not so bright, hot, or loud as to upset the patient.

Last, but not least, they offered a version of palliative care based on medical efforts to make the terminal stage of illness more comfortable through the use of patent remedies based on opium. Like late twentieth-century hospice advocates, Victorian physicians were keenly aware of the value of pain management for the terminally ill. In 1846, the German doctor C. W. Hufeland declared his enthusiasm for the use of opium for the dying, remarking on its capacity to soothe pain but also clear the mind and improve a patient's mood. Physicians agreed with Hufeland that the goal was not to drug dying patients into a stupor. The patients least wracked with pain were those who were best able to withstand the thought of their approaching demise and experience "an easy, calm, and collected death."[23] Hufeland and his German medical colleague Carl Marx were emphatic that narcotics should be used only to relieve pain, not hasten death. They tended to oppose placing these remedies in the hands of patients themselves, a clear indication that they opposed assisted suicide as a solution to the dying process. To Hufeland, it was not up to the doctor to decide whether the patient was "happy or unhappy, worthwhile or not." Should the doctor make these decisions, "the consequences would be unforeseeable and the doctor could well become the most dangerous person in the state."[24]

WILLIAM MUNK

The medical community's combination of moral support and effective use of opiates dovetailed with a consensus among nineteenth-century physicians that, when death was imminent, all thoughts of trying to prolong the patient's life with aggressive curative attempts should be banished. There was nothing terribly new about such thinking; Francis Bacon (as we have seen) had voiced it centuries earlier. Some nineteenth-century physicians even believed that they were at their best when they were ministering to the dying. Englishman William Munk's *Euthanasia* (1887) made this very point. Munk (1816–1898) defined euthanasia as a "calm and easy death."[25] He claimed that, in his experience, the "approaches to death are so gentle, and the act of dying so easy, that nature herself provides a perfect euthanasia." Like his American counterpart, the renowned physician Jacob Bigelow, Munk took a conservative approach to therapeutics and emphasized instead the palliation of disease. As long as there was proper medical care, there was no need to speed up death to relieve suffering.

Munk concurred with Hufeland's theory about the judicious use of opium, but he also paid particular attention to the value of religious faith for the terminally ill. "A firm belief in the mercy of God" made it easier to die a calm and comfortable death. "Disbelievers," according to Munk, tended to be more anxious on their deathbeds than believers, and thus died so uncomfortably that they often made a classical euthanasia impossible.[26] The typicality of Munk's opinions might be questioned in light of his conversion to Roman Catholicism at age twenty-six, but they were basically consistent with his clinical conviction that mental rather than physical anguish caused the worst distress in the dying patient. Many of Munk's nineteenth-century medical colleagues, including noted surgeon Benjamin Brodie, viewed matters in the same way.

Thus, the way nineteenth-century palliative-care doctors interpreted euthanasia was highly dissimilar to the way euthanasia is most often defined today. Doctors in the nineteenth century prided themselves on recognizing the moment when care for the chronically ill should switch from cure to consolation and pain management. They tended to be suspicious of what had passed for standard therapy up to their time, the frequent bloodlettings and purgatives employed by their predecessors, and advocated a more cautious approach to treatment. "Do no harm" became their slogan, and this especially applied to the dying patient who deserved comfort rather than aggressive efforts to cure.

Because nineteenth-century healers possessed nothing remotely resembling the life-prolonging machinery of modern medicine, their ethical dilemmas were not exactly the same as those confronted by their present-day successors. Nineteenth-century doctors were not faced with the spectacle, all too evident today, of dying or permanently unconscious patients being kept alive by respirators and feeding machines. But, by the same token, it is difficult to imagine that a doctor such as Munk would have been an advocate of active mercy killing even if he had had at his disposal the medical technology of today. Munk knew fully what the options were for dying people. He knew that other doctors sometimes surreptitiously hastened the deaths of patients. He knew that many deaths did not measure up to the standards he set for euthanasia. Yet he also sensed that, in raising the issue of euthanasia, the medical profession was in a delicate position, poised between enriching a long-standing tradition in palliative treatment and embarking on clinical voyages into an ethical unknown. Despite all the changes in medicine since Munk's time, this basic ethical dilemma remains the same to the present day.

Munk's and Hufeland's views about what constituted the good death were fairly typical of their generation. But they also coincided with the waning of the Evangelical spirit in the late nineteenth century, bringing to a close an epoch in the history of euthanasia. Their interpretations of a good death were the last eloquent and compassionate echoes of a model of euthanasia that stretched back as far as the late Middle Ages. Though few realized it at the time, the gradual secularization of Western society was steadily creating a scepticism more powerful than that of the Enlightenment about traditional religious paradigms concerning not just death, but also birth, sexuality, and reproduction. By the early decades of the twentieth century, a different understanding of euthanasia was becoming increasingly popular. It harked back both to the Enlightenment with its celebration of personal autonomy and the superiority of scientific knowledge, and to the pre-Christian, ancient form of euthanasia that included tolerance of infanticide, mercy killing, and assisted suicide. Yet, it was also inspired by the new, revolutionary theories of eugenics and Darwinist biology. As these varieties of scientific naturalism rose in popularity, Munk's theory of euthanasia swiftly became a footnote to history.

NOTES

1. Samuel E. Sprott, *The English Debate on Suicide from Donne to Hume* (Lasalle, Ind.: Open Court, 1961), 94.

2. Georges Minois, *History of Suicide: Voluntary Death in Western Culture*, trans. Lydia G. Cochrane (Baltimore: Johns Hopkins University Press, 1999), 180–181.

3. Minois, *History of Suicide*, 184.

4. Harold Nicolson, *The Age of Reason (1700–1789)* (London: Panther Books, 1968), 369–370.

5. Erwin H. Ackerknecht, "Death in the History of Medicine," *Bulletin of the History of Medicine* 42 (1968): 19–23, 21.

6. Minois, *History of Suicide*, 228, 234.

7. Minois, *History of Suicide*, 251.

8. Minois, *History of Suicide*, 230.

9. Minois, *History of Suicide*, 254.

10. Lester G. Crocker, "The Discussion of Suicide in the Eighteenth Century," *Journal of the History of Ideas* 13 (1952): 72.

11. Jacques Barzun, *From Dawn to Decadence: 500 Years of Western Cultural Life* (New York: HarperCollins, 2000), 472–473.

12. Nicolson, *The Age of Reason*, 511.

13. Minois, *History of Suicide*, 218.

14. David E. Stannard, "Death and Dying in Puritan New England," *American Historical Review* 78 (1973): 1309.

15. James A. Morone, *Hellfire Nation: The Politics of Sin in American History* (New Haven: Yale University Press, 2002), 284.

16. Pat Jalland, *Death in the Victorian Family* (New York: Oxford University Press, 1996), 20.

17. Jalland, *Death in the Victorian Family*, 168–169.

18. John T. McGreevy, *Catholicism and American Freedom: A History* (New York: Norton, 2003), 28.

19. Lewis O. Saum, "Death in the Popular Mind of Pre–Civil War America," in *Death in America*, ed. David E. Stannard (Philadelphia: University of Pennsylvania Press, 1975), 32–33.

20. Kenneth M. Ludmerer, *Learning to Heal: The Development of American Medical Education* (New York: Basic, 1985), 9.

21. Saum, "Death in the Popular Mind of Pre–Civil War America," 47.

22. Jalland, *Death in the Victorian Family*, 85.

23. William Munk, *Euthanasia: Or, Medical Treatment in Aid of an Easy Death* (New York: Arno Press, 1977, reprint of 1887 ed.), 23.

24. Michael Burleigh, *Death and Deliverance: "Euthanasia" in Germany, 1900–1945* (Cambridge: Cambridge University Press, 1994), 12.

25. Munk, *Euthanasia*, 5.

26. Munk, *Euthanasia*, 23.

3

METHOD OF ESCAPE

Just when it appeared that the traditional definition of a good death was gaining renewed vigor, the history of euthanasia changed direction abruptly. Beginning in the late nineteenth century, and continuing to the present day, society has increasingly interpreted euthanasia to mean actual mercy killing or medically assisted suicide. The preconditions for such a shift already existed in the nineteenth century. By the turn of the twentieth century, the ability of organized medicine to alleviate pain, diagnose disease, and predict its future course was so formidable that doctors were becoming powerful authority figures in the death chamber. At the same time, some members of the medical profession were actually hastening the deaths of patients with drug overdoses. But virtually no physician before the middle of the nineteenth century advocated the practice publicly. Before doctors or anyone else could take this momentous step, it was necessary that the cultural climate change in ways that would tolerate the open discussion of what qualified as a life worth living. Such a dramatic shift did indeed begin to occur after mid-century, triggering a debate over the value of human life that would peak on the eve of World War II, just as Nazi Germany began implementing a program that would see thousands of human beings put to death because their lives were deemed worthless. This human tragedy continued to cast a long shadow over the history of euthanasia at the dawn of the twenty-first century.

A NEW DEFINITION OF EUTHANASIA

If one event signaled the starting point of the modern history of euthanasia, it was an article published in 1870 by an obscure schoolteacher named

Samuel D. Williams. Published in the *Essays* of the equally obscure Birmingham Speculative Club in England, Williams's article quickly became the most influential defense of active euthanasia or mercy killing since classical antiquity. It was published in the heyday of England's scholarly periodicals, a time when magazines of high intellectual quality were read avidly by an increasingly educated audience.[1] Over the next three years, Williams's article was quoted at length and favorably reviewed in a variety of journals. Significantly, Williams did not belong to the medical profession, further proof that the debate over euthanasia historically has had less to do with medical practice than with tectonic shifts in public attitudes toward the value of human life.

In advocating voluntary active euthanasia and physician-assisted suicide, Williams was instrumental in redefining euthanasia as an act of mercy killing rather than a passive process in which the discomforts of death are mitigated but not intentionally ended by painkillers. Harking back to Seneca, the ancient Roman writer and defender of suicide, Williams rehearsed many of the Enlightenment arguments in favor of the freedom to take one's own life. But what made his speech revolutionary was his bold proposal that a new conception of "worthwhile" life should replace the old doctrine that all human life was sacred.

His justifications for this major shift included the accusation that Christian society was hypocritical when it denounced euthanasia as murder and yet executed criminals and willingly risked the lives of thousands of young men in wartime. He also attacked the "double effect" theory of indirect euthanasia, which Roman Catholic ethicists would later deploy in their opposition to legalizing active euthanasia. The use of morphine and other drugs to relieve pain, even if it shortened a patient's life, has long been considered ethical, and was thought to be so in Williams's day. As the editors of the *Lancet* wrote in 1899, physicians were "perfectly justified in pushing such treatment to an extreme degree, if that is the only way of affording freedom from acute suffering. . . . [W]e are of the opinion that even should death result the medical man has done the best he can for his patient."[2] But to Williams, there was no fundamental difference between intentionally administering drugs to put patients out of their misery and administering painkillers with the knowledge that doing so might end the patient's life. Doctors who did the latter and ended up killing their patients were simply performing a version of mercy killing. Why, he asked, were there so many objections to lethal doses for "hopelessly suffering" and dying patients who begged to be released from their agony?

Yet Williams was not content to simply ask pertinent questions that bioethicists are still grappling with at the beginning of the twenty-first century. He wanted to jettison ages-old doctrines about the sanctity of human life. Time and again, he argued that the "mortal struggle" that takes place in nature had no respect for human beings. Those who perished due to illness, disability, or old age were merely succumbing to the fate of all "weak" creatures who lost out to the "hardiest" individuals. Williams had a difficult time imagining a more compassionate act than painlessly ending the lives of these unfortunate, suffering people.

Essayist, rationalist philosopher, and Balliol graduate Lionel Tollemache quickly added his voice to the fledgling pro-euthanasia camp by backing Williams's rejection of a theological definition of mercy killing. Tollemache preferred to view euthanasia from a social or utilitarian perspective. He argued that people who were "unhealthy, unhappy, and useless" should choose assisted suicide because their death, besides being a compassionate solution, meant more resources for productive members of society. Tollemache insisted that euthanasia should be purely voluntary, but critics pointed out that denying the same compassion and social calculus to the nonconsenting (the mentally ill, for example) was hardly consistent. How long could society hold the line, Tollemache's opponents asked, before the sick and "useless" who refused to commit suicide were deemed to be selfish by impatient fellow citizens?[3]

Williams's and Tollemache's social justifications of euthanasia sparked a brief reaction among physicians on both sides of the Atlantic Ocean. A handful of doctors admitted to actual mercy killing, but the overwhelming consensus within the profession was that "in the present state of society, the practice of Euthanasia was illegal, and could only be regarded as the practice of murder." The prestigious *Boston Medical and Surgical Journal* (later the *New England Journal of Medicine*) made the crucial distinction between "active" and "passive" euthanasia when it endorsed the voluntary refusal to use heroic, extreme methods to keep dying patients alive simply to prolong their lives. There was a world of difference between letting nature take its course and actually shortening patients' lives through medical intervention. "It is equally criminal to accelerate by one hour the death of a person as to cause it," uttered a British professor of legal medicine in 1882.[4]

This debate, played out in the pages of the leading medical journals of the late nineteenth century, illustrated how the word "euthanasia" was rapidly gaining its modern-day connotation as an act of hastening death. It also demonstrated clearly that the medical profession feared advocating the legalization of euthanasia lest it create the perception that the physician was ready to "don the robes of an executioner," as a *Journal of the American Medical Association* editorial put it in 1885.[5]

THE DARWINIST REVOLUTION

Even as the medical profession balked at supporting a "quick and painless death" for terminally ill patients who requested it, powerful challenges to orthodox views on the sanctity of life were already underway in the late nineteenth century. Radical theories of natural history were enjoying mounting popularity among literate society. The most famous interpretation of natural history to explode onto the Victorian scene was Charles Darwin's theory of evolution according to natural selection. But other concepts such as eugenics and the theory of degeneracy also grew rapidly in popularity as the nineteenth century drew to a close. Their cumulative effect was to strengthen the belief that, in Samuel Williams's words, nature "knows nothing" about the sacredness of human life. In a stunning turn of events, late nineteenth-century society was confronted with an all-embracing scientific theory that seemed to subvert cardinal moral principles about the nature of human life that dated back to the earliest centuries of Christianity. That these same principles were shared by other major faiths around the world made the coming of Darwinism a revolutionary event and a critical crossroads in human history.

Darwinism, the belief that biological species have evolved over long stretches of time due to the action of purely natural causes, made its first appearance with the publication of Darwin's *Origin of Species* (1859). Naturalist views about evolution, such as the theory of the inheritance of acquired characteristics that was developed by Jean-Baptiste Lamarck (1744–1829), had been around for decades by the time Charles Darwin (1809–1882) dared to go public with his ideas. But the *Origin of Species* introduced a new and attractive explanation for the world's immense diversity of flora and fauna. Darwin, using data that he had gathered during his voyage on the *Beagle* (1831–1836), and inspired by his reading of Thomas Malthus's *Essay on the Principle of Population* (1798), hypothesized that, throughout natural history, species were modified because the fittest individuals survived the fierce struggle for existence over nature's limited food supply. Those that survived tended to transmit their favored traits through heredity more often than supposedly "unfit" individuals, thus accounting for the changes species underwent over time. Darwin called the whole process "natural selection," claiming it dispensed with the need to invoke the special creation of species by God.

More daring was *The Descent of Man* (1871), in which Darwin contended that all human life had descended from one primitive ancestor, meaning that the human race was not created in the likeness of God. Just as shocking was his firm message that the human mind and all its powers—intelligence, reason, artistic creativity, moral instincts—were purely the products of natural evolution. In other words, the attributes of the human soul were historically contingent. From the Darwinist perspective, human life was inherently no more valuable than any other natural form of life.

Darwinism not only called into question the immutability of human morality and the existence of a soul. It helped to foster belief in the theory of degeneracy. The theory of degeneracy actually predated the *Origin of Species*, having been formulated by the French physician Benedict-Augustin Morel (1809–1871) in 1857.[6] Morel and his followers often disagreed about the particular details of the theory of degeneracy, but they all believed that the human race was in severe danger of becoming less biologically robust as time went on. After studying how Europe's teeming millions of poor people lived, degeneracy theorists argued that the laws of heredity ensured that pathological traits such as alcoholism and mental illness, once acquired, could be inherited by later generations and lead to the deterioration or extinction of racial stock. If Darwin's theory of evolution according to natural selection accounted for the progressive development of species, degeneracy theory had a much gloomier message: evolution could go backward as well as forward.

The specter of degeneration due to heredity haunted Darwin. In *The Descent of Man*, he worried about how modern medicine, hospitals, asylums, and other charitable institutions affected evolution. Because they essentially protected society's unfit from the blind ruthlessness of natural selection, they enabled the weak and improvident to survive and reproduce their own kind. Meanwhile, the tax-paying, hard-working, thrifty, sober, law-abiding classes tended to do the responsible thing and have smaller families than the "reckless, degraded, and vicious" members of society. To Darwin and his many admirers, the fertility gap between fit and unfit was widening as time went on, leaving civilization in deep trouble. Although he offered no concrete policy recommendations to address this alarming differential birthrate, Darwin clearly wished to see the fertility of the lower social ranks seriously curtailed. If not, he predicted anxiously, the fit classes would be swamped by the less fit and degeneration would rule.

Darwin recoiled at the thought that coercive measures were necessary to stem the tide of degeneration. But his followers were not as shy. The link between euthanasia and Darwin's theory prompted one American doctor to remark in 1879 that "euthanasia was as sure to be accepted as was the doctrine of evolution."[7] Williams and Tollemache were just two of many figures who in the years after *The Descent of Man* methodically applied Darwinist concepts to society in order to justify legalizing euthanasia. They reasoned that if social welfare programs protected the sick and disabled from "nature red in tooth and claw" (as the poet Tennyson described it in 1850), then society was perfectly entitled to end their lives painlessly before they posed a threat to the evolution of the species. By ordering euthanasia for these groups, society was simply doing what nature did ordinarily, yet in a civilized, humane, and compassionate manner.

EUGENICS

Darwin's pessimistic thoughts about the disastrous possibilities of heredity were shared by many of his late Victorian contemporaries, including his cousin Francis Galton. Beginning in the 1860s, Galton wrote copiously about the need to boost the birthrate of society's best and brightest. In 1883, he coined the term "eugenics" to refer to these and other efforts to improve the biological quality of future generations. Eugenics, often defined as the science of human breeding, could be either positive or negative. Positive eugenics included proposals to persuade the fit classes to have large families, such as selective family allowances. Negative eugenics consisted of policies that would prevent the unfit from reproducing their own kind, including sterilization programs targeting people with disabilities. "What nature does blindly, slowly, ruthlessly, man may do providently, quickly, and kindly," Galton asserted.[8]

Galton made no secret of the fact that in promoting eugenics he was engaged in a frontal attack on traditional religion. A pious disposition, Galton suspected, was itself a hereditary trait. His goal was to make eugenics into "a new religion" that rendered the mainline churches obsolete. Later admirers of Galton agreed. The noted Irish playwright and critic George Bernard Shaw observed in 1905 that "there is no reasonable excuse for refusing to face the fact that nothing but a eugenic religion can save our civilization."[9]

Eugenics caught on like few other ideas in modern history. Adherents of eugenics plainly viewed it as a way of addressing Darwin's own foreboding about civilized society's tendency to thwart the effects of natural selection. Eugenic organizations were founded in Europe, Canada, the United States, and Latin America. Colleges, universities, and public schools taught the principles of eugenics. Biology textbooks accepted eugenics as scientific truth. Liberal pastors, inspired by the Social Gospel message of reforming earthly conditions as a way of saving the world, preached eugenics from their pulpits.[10] In the name of eugenics, governments around the world ordered the building of custodial institutions for the handicapped, the sterilization of mental patients, the biological inspection of immigrants, and the medical screening of marriage partners. The most notorious example of a government putting eugenic ideas into practice was Nazi Germany's 1933 law permitting the forcible sterilization of alcoholics, epileptics, the insane, and the mentally retarded. By the time war broke out in 1939, 400,000 Germans had been sterilized according to the Nazi law. Yet eugenic sterilization programs also flourished in Progressive-era America and social-democratic Sweden, while enjoying the support of many socialists, liberals, conservationists, birth-control activists, and women's rights advocates around the world. An English political radical exclaimed in 1917 that "unless the socialist is a eugenicist as well, the socialist state will speedily perish from racial degradation."[11]

Eugenics declined in popularity after World War II when the news about Hitler's sterilization law convinced many that eugenics was Nazi science. But in the meantime, eugenics proved to be one of the most influential social movements in modern history. Among other things, eugenics encouraged open discussion about which lives were more valuable than others and thus helped to smooth the social acceptance of euthanasia in the twentieth century.

The cumulative impact of Darwinism, eugenics, and degeneracy theories was a widespread debate over the value of human life. As Williams stated, "it may well be doubted if life have any sacredness about it, apart from the use made of it by its possessor . . . and, indeed, seeing that life is so transitory a thing . . . it is hard to understand the meaning of the word 'sacred' when applied to it. . . . Life is a thing to be used freely and sacrificed freely."[12] Stripped of its religious connotations, life suddenly was subject to a utilitarian, biological calculus in the eyes of eugenicists and Darwinists. To them, some lives counted more than others. This was precisely what supporters of euthanasia wanted to hear. There were no better rationales for advocating mercy killing than eugenics and Darwinism.

ROBERT INGERSOLL

Admiration for Darwinism led lawyer Robert Ingersoll (1833–1899) to construct one of the first American justifications for a right to euthanasia.

Born in Dresden, New York, Ingersoll traveled the length and breadth of the country after the Civil War, lecturing against conventional religion before sold-out (and often raucous) crowds. He first came to national prominence in 1876 when, at the Republican National Convention in Cincinnati, he nominated James G. Blaine for president, but the delegates chose Rutherford B. Hayes instead. In his day, Ingersoll was known as "The Great Agnostic," defending such unpopular causes as birth control, racial tolerance, and women's rights. A latter-day admirer argues that Ingersoll was "the first American to lay out a coherent secular humanist alternative" to traditional religion. His critics, on the other hand, dubbed him "Robert Injuresoul."[13] The nineteenth century was "Darwin's century," in Ingersoll's view, and in trying to fight Darwinism, Christianity was obstructing the march of truth. Christian beliefs had to give way before the teachings of evolutionary theory, he announced. "The survival of the fittest," Ingersoll maintained, "does away with original sin."

In 1894, Ingersoll created a great stir when he argued that a person "being slowly devoured by cancer" should enjoy the "right to end his pain and pass through happy sleep to dreamless rest." No God could take pleasure, Ingersoll contended, in the suffering of such people. Medical ethics needed to be reformed when it came to death and dying, Ingersoll concluded. He added that morality "is the best thing to do under the circumstances" and depended on the situation facing each individual. Yet, utilitarianism also informed Ingersoll's approach to ethical conduct. The "best thing to do under the circumstances" was determined less by personal choice than by "that which will increase the sum of human happiness—or lessen it the least."

In his advocacy of euthanasia, Ingersoll drew inspiration from other scientific sources than Darwinism. Ingersoll was one of many nineteenth-century liberals (including English philosopher John Stuart Mill) who borrowed heavily from the theories of the French philosopher Auguste Comte (1798–1857). Comte was the founder of positivism, the belief that societies evolved through three stages of development. The first stage was the theological one, when people attributed all natural phenomena to the gods. The second was the metaphysical stage, when people ceased invoking gods and instead believed in abstract theories. The third was the positivist stage, during which individuals would increasingly rely on empirical explanations based on rigorous observation and the mathematical laws that governed the world. Comte contended that the nineteenth century would usher in the positivist stage. Equipped with such scientific knowledge, Comte predicted society would be able to harness these laws for the prosperity and progress of the human race. Scientists in the positivist age, according to Comte, would be the natural leaders of society.

Ingersoll maintained that the founder of positivism would be "lovingly remembered as a benefactor of the human race." Ingersoll was like other liberals, including sociologist E. A. Ross and clergyman Charles Potter, two Americans who in coming years would translate their respect for positivism into support for eugenics and euthanasia. Positivism's veneration of science also encouraged Comte's followers to embrace Darwinism. Similarly, positivism's celebration of progress and social reorganization, as well as its assault on superstition and sterile metaphysics, appealed to liberals who had confidence in reform, government interventionism, and the competence of experts.[14]

SECULARIZATION

The rise of Darwinism, eugenics, and positivism coincided with the broader trend of secularization that was sweeping industrialized nations in the late nineteenth century. Defined by historian Owen Chadwick as the "growing tendency in mankind to do without religion, or to try to do without religion," secularization refers to the process by which religious ideas and institutions lose their public significance. Symptoms of secularization in England became particularly prominent in 1860–1880, including the "willingness of devout men to meet un-devout men in society and to honor them for their sincerity instead of condemning them for their lack of faith."[15]

Another symptom of secularization in the late Victorian era was the mounting popularity of Darwinist models and metaphors for explaining how society functioned. This current fostered trust in both science and scientists to make sense of the world even at the expense of religious teachings. Books such as John William Draper's *History of the Conflict between Science and Religion* (1874) and Andrew Dickson White's *A History of the Warfare of Science with Theology in Christendom* (1896), which tended to depict the churches as perennial obstacles to science, reason, progress, and enlightenment, accelerated secularization by encouraging people to choose science over religion.

A third symptom was the waning of the Evangelical movement in Anglo-American society by the 1870s. As it receded, many people began looking for sources of authority other than religion. It was no accident that the word "secularization" was coined in the 1860s, at roughly the same time the terms "clericalism" and "anti-clericalism" first came into use. Secularization as a diffuse cultural trend was closely linked to the late nineteenth-century protests against the influence of the Roman Catholic clergy over mass mores, especially in Catholic countries such as France, Belgium, and Italy.

By challenging the authority of church teaching, secularization subtly altered the way in which some people thought about death. Some no longer viewed the torment and general suffering of dying patients as an experience to be endured stoically and piously. Increasingly, people perceived death to be a medical event that could be alleviated by ether, chloroform, or morphine. To some, that included administering overdoses to terminally ill patients.

Secularization, like Darwinism and other naturalist theories, did not necessarily cause devout people to turn into atheists. Many late Victorian Darwinists had already begun to question their faith before they became evolutionists. Some saw no necessary contradiction between religious faith and belief in evolution. But the result was the same: by the dawn of the Edwardian period, many members of the respectable classes agreed with liberals such as John Stuart Mill that individual freedom of thought trumped obedience to church dogma. As one historian has written, "the Victorian father goes to church. The Edwardian son stays at home."[16] Or the son joined a more liberal and seemingly rationalist church that better suited his heart and mind, such as the Unitarians.

UNITARIANISM AND ETHICAL CULTURE

The theological roots of Unitarianism can be traced back to sixteenth-century Europe, where various religious reformers rejected the doctrine of the Trinity, claiming that a single God was more consistent with the scriptures. Unitarian ideas came to North America from Britain in the seventeenth century. Unitarianism gathered momentum in eighteenth-century America as a religious backlash to the austere Calvinist teachings of New England Puritanism. Countless Christians chafed under the grim message that only a few were saved by God's grace and most were doomed to damnation. Emphasizing God's benevolence, human free will, and the dignity rather than the depravity of human nature, preachers in the late eighteenth century and early nineteenth century called for a more liberal and rational theology. Noted Americans such as Thomas Jefferson and the British-born scientist (and discoverer of oxygen) Joseph Priestley embraced Unitarian teaching. By the mid-nineteenth century, many Puritan Congregational churches had begun calling themselves Unitarian. Yet the American Unitarian Association (founded in 1825) remained a relatively small church; by 1900, there were fewer than 100,000 Unitarians in the United States.

As the new religion spread throughout the nineteenth century, it became more and more liberal in the process. Unitarians increasingly stressed the importance of individualism and the need to question orthodox Christian doctrine. By the turn of the twentieth century, Unitarians were highly sceptical about biblical authority and even the divinity of Christ. The Social Gospel, with its emphasis on reforming the social and economic conditions of this world, became a central tenet of Unitarianism. Duty to the less fortunate rather than adherence to accepted dogma was the chief teaching of early twentieth-century Unitarians, who believed that individuals developed themselves fully when they dedicated themselves to social service. Unitarianism expressed the longing of liberal Christians to break free from what they thought were the sterile moral prohibitions of the established churches and create a new morality that more closely conformed to the needs of individual human beings. Unitarians' optimistic willingness to overthrow traditional religious value systems explains why so many of them flocked to the euthanasia movement in the twentieth century.

Besides Unitarianism, another religion that the Edwardian son might have joined instead of his father's church was Ethical Culture, founded in 1876 by the German-born American theologian Felix Adler (1851–1933). Ethical Culture and Unitarianism proved to be the religions most supportive of the legalization of euthanasia. In fact, Unitarianism and Ethical Culture shared some historical roots: shortly after the U.S. Civil War, Adler played a leading role in a small group that had broken away from Unitarianism.[17] Trained as a rabbi, Adler turned his back on Judaism and decided to construct a religion that rejected doctrine and personalized ethics. Adler preached that ethical decisions should never be based on absolute principles but must be tailored to fit the distinctive circumstances surrounding each individual's life. Adler constructed Ethical Culture as an eclectic religion that he hoped Jews and Christians could accept. When it came to suicide, Adler maintained that patients dying in pain and unhappiness had a right to request from their physicians "a cup of relief" to end their lives. He urged that euthanasia be legalized, safeguarded, and purely voluntary. But his enthusiasm for the notion that the value of individual life was conditioned by changing circumstances fit what Darwinism and other naturalist theories were saying about the contingent nature of human life. To Adler, mercy killing and assisted suicide were not necessarily taboo if they suited the needs of certain individuals. Adler contended that it was up to individuals to decide if they wanted euthanasia. Yet, philosophically, he had a difficult time distinguishing what a person might choose to do and what a person ought to do.

In fashioning a self-consciously religious justification for euthanasia, Adler and Ethical Culture, along with numerous Unitarians, posed a more long-term threat to orthodox theories of the value of human life than Darwinism. Opponents of Darwinism could always argue that it was merely a scientific theory and that, until it was completely proven, there was no pressing need to revamp conventional morality to fit its tenets. Yet Adler's "practical religion" and its defense of mercy killing made it more difficult for leaders of established churches to maintain that all religion taught that euthanasia was a grievous sin.

Ethical Culture found its way back to Germany, where the German Society for Ethical Culture was founded in 1892. Since then, it has proved to be a breeding ground for support of legalized euthanasia in Germany, the United States, and elsewhere. But in the short term, the main forces behind the growth of support for euthanasia in imperial Germany (1871–1918) were Darwinism and eugenics. There, and in other Western countries, some naturalists argued that acceptance of Darwinist evolution as a scientific theory did not change traditional ethics and customary attitudes toward euthanasia, or for that matter suicide, abortion, infanticide, birth control, and sexual morality. German philosophers who followed the teachings of the late eighteenth-century thinker Immanuel Kant contended that the natural sciences were separate from the human sciences, and thus should not be applied to the study of social, religious, or ethical issues. However, their voices were often drowned out by the bold assertions of prominent German scientists who insisted that Darwinism constituted an entirely new philosophy of life with revolutionary consequences for the meaning and value of life.

ERNST HAECKEL

The advocacy of Darwinism, eugenics, and euthanasia in German society up to World War I can be traced back to the life and career of scientist Ernst Haeckel (1834–1919). Haeckel was a self-proclaimed popularizer of Darwinism, adherent to eugenics, and proponent of euthanasia. Beginning in the 1860s, Haeckel preached the virtues of Darwinism as a new worldview that would liberate human beings from the supposed thrall of Judeo-Christian tyranny. In 1900, he helped to sponsor the Krupp Prize Competition for the best book-length answer to the question: "what do we learn from the principles of biological evolution in regard to domestic political developments and legislation of states?" The winner was the social Darwinist physician Wilhelm Schallmayer, who in 1891 had published the first explicitly eugenic book in German history. Six years later, Haeckel founded the Monist League, an organization dedicated to spreading the gospel of social Darwinism and combating the influence of Christianity. On the eve of World War I, a majority of members within the Monist League came out in support of legalizing euthanasia.

Haeckel's efforts, reaching well beyond Germany to the English-speaking world, were based on the belief that the interests of the species always came before those of the individual. "The individual with his personal existence," a youthful Haeckel wrote in 1864, "appears to me only a temporary member in this large chain, as a rapidly vanishing vapor. . . . Personal individual existence appears to me so horribly miserable, petty, and worthless, that I see it as intended for nothing but for destruction." The death of the individual, wrote another German social Darwinist in 1889, "is the condition of life for the whole."[18]

The view that the welfare of the group was more important than individual life explains why Haeckel and other German Darwinists were in favor of enacting both eugenic and euthanasia laws around the turn of the twentieth century. August Forel, a leading psychiatrist, Wilhelm Schallmayer, winner of the 1900 Krupp Prize Competition, and Alfred Ploetz, organizer of the Society for Race Hygiene, the first eugenics society in history, all boldly questioned the Christian prohibition on killing innocent life. Not all German eugenicists supported legalizing euthanasia, but few adamantly disagreed with Haeckel's defense of suicide, the ancient Spartan practice of murdering weak and sickly infants, or Forel's advocacy of mercy killing the mentally and physically handicapped. By the 1930s, many concurred with the Darwinist opinion of Alfred Hoche, professor of psychiatry at the University of Freiburg, who wrote in his memoirs that "the continued existence of the species is everything, the individual is nothing."[19] Hoche co-authored perhaps the most influential pro-euthanasia book in pre–World War II German history, *Permitting the Destruction of Life Unworthy of Life* (1920).

Sentiments such as these within the German scientific and medical communities revealed that, as the twentieth century dawned, the issue of mercy killing in only a few short years had gone from being a topic virtually no one dared to support openly to a subject that enjoyed a small but vocal backing. This tiny, pro-euthanasia minority did not dream for a moment that overnight it could convert public opinion or even medical opinion to approval of any form of euthanasia, whether voluntary or involuntary. But this group's exertions meant it was now possible to broach the topic of euthanasia in polite, educated society. The taboo against taking innocent life, not just the prohibition against suicide, had been questioned by leading individuals in highly respected professions at a time when science enjoyed a lofty cultural profile. They had questioned the taboo against murdering innocent life both in terms of individual rights and the interests of society at large. As the Western world began to enter the age of twentieth-century mass politics, with its ritualistic celebration of the nation, the secular state, and personal liberties enshrined in a written constitution, proponents of euthanasia would discover a growing audience for their message of liberation, freedom, and national efficiency.

ANNIE BESANT

Darwinists, eugenicists, and followers of Ethical Culture were not the only allies that euthanasia advocates could count on around the turn of the twentieth century. As the movement in favor of expanding women's rights gained momentum in the waning years of the nineteenth century, a handful of social reformers began arguing that the legalization of euthanasia was as desirable as the liberalization of birth control, divorce, and property laws, as well as voting rights and greater access to the professions and educational institutions for women. Euthanasia as a social reform had special meaning for women. Women knew firsthand the acute pain (and sometimes tragic death) of childbirth and were subject to a variety of harrowing terminal diseases of the breast and pelvic organs, until twentieth-century advances in surgery and medicine began to make a significant difference in women's experience of these conditions.[20] Moreover, women were more likely than men to undertake the care of the sick and dying as a normal part of their nurturing role in the family. Similarly, women tended to live longer than men, which meant they had more opportunities to witness the death of loved ones and faced the prospect of dying alone while depending on the charity of strangers for their care. The inclusion of euthanasia among the host of reforms sought by women activists would become much more apparent in the twentieth century. But one nineteenth-century pioneer who blazed the trail for others to follow was Englishwoman Annie Besant (1847–1933).

Besant is best known as a feminist who tirelessly campaigned to make birth control legal in Britain. In 1877, she was a co-defendant with Charles Bradlaugh in a sensational trial that gripped the attention of English polite society. Besant and Bradlaugh were charged with obscenity for disseminating information about contraception. Besant was sentenced to six months in prison, but the verdict was overturned on a technicality.

A member of the socialist Fabian Society and England's National Secular Society, Besant preached free love and late in life helped to start the Indian nationalist movement. She was heavily influenced by Darwinism and the theories of economist Thomas Malthus (1766–1834), who argued that population growth tended to outstrip food production. Malthus concluded that this ratio between population and food supply meant the human race would endure famine, plague, and other miseries unless people voluntarily limited the size of their families. Besant believed that the Malthusian trap could be avoided through artificial contraception. Her neo-Malthusian alarmism led her to loudly echo Darwin's fears about racial degeneration. She passionately urged eugenic policies to curb the fertility of Europe's teeming urban masses, who, in the words of fellow Fabian George Bernard Shaw, supposedly bred "like rabbits."

None of these views was inconsistent with Besant's feminism: she believed state-run eugenic measures were necessary because on them depended women's emancipation from what she called "the radically false notion of 'woman's sphere.' " In her attacks on the so-called "cult of domesticity," Besant anticipated later twentieth-century feminists who argued that birth control, by freeing women from unwanted pregnancies, enabled them to make contributions to society outside as well as inside the home. If some women were unable to see that bringing unfit or excess children into the world was both a "sin against society" and contrary to their own interests as human beings, then Besant believed their "reckless multiplication" had to be stopped forcibly. Thanks to Besant's Darwinism, socialism, eugenicism, and neo-Malthusianism, her views on euthanasia were decidedly authoritarian. She utterly rejected the notion that life was a gift from God. An individual's life was the "property of the state," she wrote, and when death beckoned, it was time for the individual to give up this property.

> The infant is nurtured, the child is educated, the man is protected by others; and in return for the life thus given, developed, preserved, society has a right to demand from its members a loyal, self-forgetting devotion to the common weal. . . . And, when we have given all we can, when strength is sinking, and life is failing, when pain racks our bodies, and the worse agony of seeing our dear ones suffer in our anguish, tortures our enfeebled minds, when the only service we can render man is to relieve him of a useless and injurious burden, then we ask that we may

be permitted to die voluntarily and painlessly, and so to crown a noble life with the laurel-wreath of a self-sacrificing death.

Clearly, Besant thought that all well-informed citizens would want to request such a "self-sacrificing death," but she also believed that it was their civic duty to do so.[21]

Besant stood out as an iconoclast in late Victorian society, a woman reformer willing to defy conventional codes of conduct. Her chief significance lies in the fact that she adumbrated later, twentieth-century trends. As that century unfolded, other women spearheading the eugenics, birth control, and abortion rights movements would follow her example and champion legalized euthanasia. Prominent female reformers such as Margaret Sanger, Charlotte Perkins Gilman, Carrie Chapman Catt, Mary Ware Dennett, Helene Stoecker, and Agnes Bluhm publicly defended the right to euthanasia while simultaneously advocating women's reproductive freedom. To these activists, the legalization of euthanasia represented important progress in the struggle for all women's rights.

THE CRISIS IN PSYCHIATRY

As various individuals increasingly dared to speak out in favor of euthanasia in the early twentieth century, a handful of physicians felt similarly bold enough to broach the topic sympathetically and publicly. American doctors were the first worldwide to admit they were asked by patients and their families to "administer some potent drug that would close the fearful struggle" (as one doctor wrote in 1873). Because American political culture stressed individual freedom of opinion and speech more than did British political culture, there was a greater American willingness to discuss euthanasia. American physicians were also the first to admit they actually put patients out of their misery with lethal injections. In 1913, one Buffalo, New York, doctor candidly declared: "I know that others have assumed the responsibility, which I myself have taken in more than one case, of producing euthanasia, when, in the terminal stage of life, a patient was suffering the tortures 'of the damned,' and has pleaded for a method of escape, the pleadings being seconded by the family."[22] These disclosures revealed nothing fundamentally new. For centuries, doctors had been ending the lives of dying patients painlessly, whether asked to or not. What was new was that a few physicians sought to exploit grim reality for propaganda purposes. They argued that because euthanasia happened anyway, the best course of action was to legalize and thus safeguard the entire process.

British physicians in favor of euthanasia were slower than their American counterparts to venture into print. The first strident English medical support for active euthanasia came in 1901 from C. E. Goddard, the medical officer of health from Willesden. Significantly, Goddard's backing of euthanasia was linked to his admiration of eugenics, which in turn grew out of the crisis in psychiatry that struck Western industrialized nations by the early twentieth century. Across Europe and North America, governments in the nineteenth century built numerous mental hospitals to house the growing population of insane people. Between 1885 and 1900, the state of Prussia expanded the number of its mental asylums from 71 to 105. In Britain, between 1847 and 1869, the number of mentally unsound inmates of public asylums increased from 5,500 to 26,867.

America experienced the same basic trends in asylum construction. In 1840, only three states had erected their own public facilities for the mentally ill. But in the 1850s, sixteen state, one federal, and four municipal asylums were opened. As time went on, however, the curative promise of the asylum dimmed. Asylum construction never seemed to catch up to the mounting rate of admissions and the declining rate of discharges. As soon as one asylum was built, another one was needed to meet demand. Existing asylums grew beyond the wildest expectations of their founders. In Paris, the world-famous and state-of-the-art Sainte-Anne asylum opened amid great fanfare in 1867 for 490 patients, but in 1911 it housed 1,100.[23] Wards quickly became overcrowded with patients suffering from chronic, incurable conditions. Psychiatrists realized that their hospitalized patients were much more difficult to treat than earlier imagined, despite the remarkable advances in medical science. "We know a lot and can do little," a German asylum doctor remarked ruefully in 1910.[24]

The most callous observers, appalled by the spectacle of handicapped patients living out their lives at state expense and without any hope of cure, sometimes suggested that it would be better for everyone concerned if these unfortunates were put out of their misery. The mentally ill were a eugenic threat to society and their lives were deemed to be "not worth living." Drawing on the analogy to the receptacle in which animals were killed painlessly with poisonous gas, a handful of physicians recommended using the "lethal chamber" for incurably handicapped patients.[25] A willingness to use the lethal chamber remained a distinctly minority position in organized medicine. Yet the day was rapidly approaching when who should not be born and who was better off dead would be acceptable questions in some professional circles.

THE AGE OF CHRONIC DISEASE

Bolstering pro-euthanasia arguments were certain facts about death and dying that had become evident by the early twentieth century. Between 1850 and 1950, mortality rates were on the decline, due primarily to public health reforms that reduced the incidence of acute, infectious diseases such as tuberculosis, measles, typhus, pneumonia, and dysentery. As the cause of death due to infectious diseases fell, the rate of mortality due to chronic diseases such as cancer rose sharply. In England and Wales, the incidence of deaths per millions from cancer went from 800 in 1900 to 1,376 in 1927. In America, the number of deaths due to cancer rose from an estimated 88,000 in 1920 to 158,000 in 1940.[26] Cancer deaths tended to be more prolonged than deaths from acute diseases, and as patients endured the pain from cancer, they and their doctors discovered that simply increasing the dosage of narcotics sometimes did not end the suffering. Too, child mortality rates were starting to drop dramatically by the early twentieth century, which meant average life expectancy was getting longer, and more and more people were dying in old age. The cumulative effect of all these trends was "the gradual move from infancy to old age as the most probable time of death." Death came to be viewed as a purely natural event caused by specific medical conditions related to aging, rather than a human tragedy cloaked in religious significance.[27]

However, this growing perception of death as an event of old age and its consequences for euthanasia were caused less by shifts in disease patterns or medical technology than by changes in sentiments regarding time-honored religious taboos. Mounting uncertainty about religious doctrine was a decisive factor in preparing the ground for the twentieth-century "discovery" of euthanasia.[28] The trauma of World War I accelerated the trend toward uncertainty about established religion and what it stood for. The wrenching spectacle of countless young men losing their lives in violent, disfiguring, dehumanizing ways in battle without opportunities for proper burial and ritualistic mourning triggered an explosion of grief that transformed accepted attitudes toward death. In the wake of World War I, secularized value systems increasingly challenged the more religious ceremonies and interpretations of the "good death."

Yet, until this uncertainty about religious teachings became genuinely deep and widespread, advocacy of euthanasia remained the minority position of radicals such as Ernst Haeckel, who complained:

> if someone would dare to make the suggestion, according to the example of the Spartans and Redskins, to kill immediately after birth the miserable and infirm children, to whom can be prophesied with assurance a sickly life, instead of preserving them to their own harm and the detriment of the whole community, our whole so-called "humane civilization" would erupt in a cry of indignation.[29]

Haeckel had no doubt that similar cries would surely erupt from organized medicine. Well into the twentieth century, the medical profession in all Western countries continued to be conservative in its moral values. Mavericks such as Goddard occasionally tried to provoke controversy by expressing their support for legalizing either voluntary or involuntary mercy killing. But rather than engender greater tolerance for euthanasia, they tended to trigger intolerance. For example, the famous Canadian clinician William Osler was only trying to be funny when he proposed in 1905 that all those over sixty years of age should be put to death with chloroform. When the predictable protests materialized in the United States, the *British Medical Journal* chided Americans for their inability to take a joke. But whether or not observers believed Osler was joking, the vast majority agreed that legalizing what was already happening at the hands of doctors and surgeons throughout America was unwise public policy. In 1906, the *British Medical Journal* noted:

> ending by what is euphemistically called euthanasia, suffering which cannot be mended, is by no means novel. Every now and again it is put forward either by literary dilettanti who discuss it as an academic subtlety, or by neurotic "intellectuals" whose high-strung temperament cannot bear the thought of pain. The medical profession has always sternly set its face against a measure that would inevitably pave the way to the grossest abuse and would degrade them to the position of executioner.[30]

As the American physician Abraham Jacobi asked rhetorically in 1912: "Would a doctor who would consent to satisfying the suggestions of the people who clamor for 'Euthanasia' ever again deserve the confidence of the public?"[31]

In fact, medical resistance to euthanasia actually gained ground around the turn of the century, thanks to the enormous progress of organized medicine. Therapeutic optimism escalated as medical scientists made discovery after discovery about the bacteriological causes of infectious diseases. Vaccines for diphtheria and syphilis were developed. Surgery was becoming safer and more successful. The first modern hospitals devoted to research and treatment were being built. Medical education in the United States was in the throes of reorganization and reform. The image of the doctor as a scientist armed with the discoveries of the laboratory steadily crystallized in the early twentieth century. The polio vaccine and penicillin, the wonder cures of the 1940s and 1950s, were still a long way off, but growing numbers of people were investing high hopes in the power of medicine to win the war against disease.

Thus, as the new century dawned, organized medicine remained resolute in its nearly unanimous condemnation of euthanasia. Medical opposition was matched by an overwhelming social consensus throughout the industrialized world that mercy killing or assisted suicide was abhorrent. But the tiny euthanasia movement had made inroads. Eugenic and Darwinist ideas enjoyed a measure of popularity in educated social circles. Simultaneously, secularization incrementally disposed people to question their religious beliefs and their churches' opposition to reforms such as birth control and sexual freedom. While public opinion appeared to be firmly anti-euthanasia, there already were social, cultural, and political currents in motion that would lead to the official founding of pro-euthanasia groups in the twentieth century.

NOTES

1. N. D. A. Kemp. *"Merciful Release": The History of the British Euthanasia Movement* (Manchester: Manchester University Press, 2002), 12. See also Christopher Kent, "Higher Journalism and the Mid-Victorian Clerisy," *Victorian Studies* 13 (1969): 181–198.

2. Ezekiel J. Emanuel, "Euthanasia: Historical, Ethical, and Empiric Perspectives," *Archives of Internal Medicine* 154 (1994): 1891.

3. Kemp, *"Merciful Release,"* 11–28.

4. W. Bruce Fye, "Active Euthanasia: An Historical Survey of Its Conceptual Origins and Introduction into Medical Thought," *Bulletin of the History of Medicine* 52 (1979): 492–502.

5. Ian Dowbiggin, *A Merciful End: The Euthanasia Movement in Modern America* (New York: Oxford University Press, 2003), 7.

6. Ian Dowbiggin, *Inheriting Madness: Professionalization and Psychiatric Knowledge in Nineteenth-Century France* (Berkeley: University of California Press, 1991).

7. Fye, "Active Euthanasia," 500.

8. Christine Rosen, *Preaching Eugenics: Religious Leaders and the American Eugenics Movement* (New York: Oxford University Press, 2004), 5.

9. Diane B. Paul, *Controlling Heredity: 1865 to the Present* (Atlantic Highlands, N.J.: Humanities Press, 1995), 75.

10. Rosen, *Preaching Eugenics.*

11. Paul, *Controlling Heredity,* 76.

12. Fye, "Active Euthanasia," 498.

13. Susan Jacoby, *Freethinkers: A History of American Secularism* (New York: Henry Holt, 2004), 158.

14. Gillis J. Harp, *Positivist Republic: Auguste Comte and the Reconstruction of American Liberalism, 1865–1920* (University Park: Pennsylvania State University Press, 1995).

15. Owen Chadwick, *The Secularization of the European Mind in the Nineteenth Century* (Cambridge: Cambridge University Press, 1975), 17, 37.

16. Chadwick, *The Secularization of the European Mind,* 6.

17. Paul K. Conkin, *American Originals: Homemade Varieties of Christianity* (Chapel Hill: University of North Carolina Press, 1997), 89.

18. Richard Weikart, "Darwinism and Death: Devaluing Human Life in Germany, 1859–1920," *Journal of the History of Ideas* 63 (2002): 329, 332.

19. Richard Weikart, *From Darwin to Hitler: Evolutionary Ethics, Eugenics, and Racism in Germany* (New York: Palgrave Macmillan, 2004), 155.

20. Edward Shorter, *A History of Women's Bodies* (New York: Basic, 1982).

21. Kemp, *"Merciful Release,"* 26.

22. Dowbiggin, *A Merciful End,* 5–6.

23. Edward Shorter, *A History of Psychiatry: From the Era of the Asylum to the Age of Prozac* (New York: Wiley, 1998), 47.

24. Roy Porter, *The Greatest Benefit to Mankind: A Medical History of Humanity* (New York: Norton, 1998), 513.

25. Russell Hollander, "Euthanasia and Mental Retardation: Suggesting the Unthinkable," *Mental Retardation* 27 (1989): 53–61; Martin A. Elks, "The 'Lethal Chamber': Further Evidence for the Euthanasia Option," *Mental Retardation* 31 (1993): 201–207.

26. James T. Patterson, *The Dread Disease: Cancer and Modern American Culture* (Cambridge, Mass.: Harvard University Press, 1987), 95.

27. Pat Jalland, *Death in the Victorian Family* (New York: Oxford University Press, 1996), 5.

28. Jalland, *Death in the Victorian Family,* 6.

29. Weikart, "Darwinism and Death," 336.

30. Dowbiggin, *A Merciful End,* 23.

31. Dowbiggin, *A Merciful End,* 6–7.

4

A HIGHER MORALITY?

The history of euthanasia in the twentieth century began much the same way it ended: in a legal experiment permitting assisted suicide. But the differences between the beginning and the end of the century could not have been greater. In the early twentieth century, there was negligible popular support anywhere for legalizing any form of euthanasia. One hundred years later, suicide had been decriminalized in many industrial societies. Public opinion polls consistently found that majorities endorsed the personal freedom to request a painless death. By the early twenty-first century, several jurisdictions on both sides of the Atlantic Ocean had enacted laws allowing either active euthanasia or assisted suicide. Courts in various countries had ruled that individuals enjoyed a right to medical aid in dying. Numerous national and international organizations advocating a right to die had also been formed. Troubling stories circulated in the media about terminally ill patients having their lives ended without their consent. These trends helped to set the stage for the conflict throughout the industrialized world over legalizing euthanasia in the early twenty-first century. Yet this struggle was firmly rooted in a series of events that stretched back to a time when social disapproval of both suicide and mercy killing was overwhelming.

TEXAS

At the beginning of the twentieth century, Texas, like all other American states, did not outlaw suicide. This legal situation dated back to the revolt of the thirteen British colonies of North America against the British monarchy at the end of the eighteenth century. U.S. statutory laws are derived from English common law, which forbade suicide because it denied the

71

king his "property" in the form of his subjects' lives. When American colonists ceased to be subjects of the British king, there was no legal justification for outlawing suicide. In 1961, Britain itself finally repealed its prohibition against suicide, but suicide in American law had long been defined legally as a private act.

Yet, no matter how Americans felt about the constitutional status of suicide, by the early twentieth century there was no indication in the United States that the absence of a legal prohibition against suicide would lead courts to rule in favor of assisted suicide. The notable exception was the Texas Court of Criminal Appeals. In 1902, it overturned the murder conviction of a physician named J. H. Grace, who had furnished his mistress with a pistol that she used to end her own life. Six years later, the same court overturned the conviction for murder of a ranch hand who had been found guilty of supplying his pregnant girlfriend with the carbolic acid she took to kill herself. The Texas court decided that there was no crime in either case because the individual performing the suicide supposedly made a rational choice to commit suicide. The person assisting in the suicide could not be guilty of a crime because, the court ruled, no crime was committed in the first place. In 1973, however, aiding or soliciting a suicide became a felony in the Lone Star State.[1]

The setting for the first suicide was a meeting of the physician, his wife, and his mistress, during which they discussed their sexual adventures. In the second case the court found that there was reason to question the motives of the ranch hand. But it still ruled that the deceased must have known fully the danger involved and thus took the poison voluntarily. People living in a later age, more sensitive to the psychological complexity surrounding suicide, and more aware of the power imbalances in gender relations, might disagree. A pregnant girlfriend ending her own life with the help of her male partner raises questions about her emotional stability and his intentions at the time of the act. Moreover, neither of these assisted suicides could be described as merciful, humane, or painless. Far from suffering with a terminal illness, the two women were young and presumably in good health. Their deaths from poisoning and gunshot wounds were anything but good deaths.

In the early twentieth century, isolated attempts to legalize euthanasia began in various states. In 1906, an effort to introduce a law permitting voluntary active euthanasia predictably went down to defeat in the Ohio state legislature by a vote of 79 to 23. The same year, a more far-reaching bill suffered a similar fate in Iowa. It called for persons with a "hopeless disease or injury and hideously deformed or idiotic children" being killed "by the administration of an anesthetic." These legislative initiatives in Ohio and Iowa accomplished little for the euthanasia movement. If they had any impact at all, it was to alert those who opposed euthanasia that more such challenges could be expected in future.

THE BLACK STORK

In 1915, a well-publicized effort to promote euthanasia was made by the American surgeon Harry Haiselden. In the early morning of November 12, a woman by the name of Anna Bollinger gave birth at the German-American Hospital in Chicago. The baby, named Allan, was somewhat deformed and suffered from a host of complications, including intestinal and rectal infirmities. As hospital chief of staff, Haiselden was called at once and consulted with the other medical staff. Spirited debate over the baby's fate ensued, but in the end, Haiselden's opinion carried the day with Allan's parents. His verdict? Deny the baby the surgery needed for it to survive.

Predictably, Allan Bollinger died several days later. By then, Haiselden was a virtual household name. After an inquest and a failed attempt to prosecute Haiselden, the Baby Bollinger story was splashed across the headlines of the nation's newspapers, thanks largely to Haiselden himself. Haiselden did not quietly "let nature complete its bungled job," as he put it. He energetically publicized his decision not to operate in the hopes that it would generate widespread support for the legalization of euthanasia for disabled persons. He wrote articles for Hearst newspapers, delivered public lectures, and posed for movie newsreels. He even helped write and star in a motion picture titled *The Black Stork*, a dramatization of the Bollinger case. When asked by a reporter about the reason behind his decision not to operate, Haiselden replied: "Eugenics? Of course, it's eugenics."[2]

Haiselden's approach chiefly derived from his deep belief in eugenics, social Darwinism, and biologically based utilitarianism. But his attitude toward the Bollinger baby was likewise shaped by his bitter hatred of institutionalization. In 1916, he published a muckraking exposé of the conditions in an Illinois home for the retarded. His fierce opposition to custodialism for the handicapped led the unmarried Haiselden to adopt two girls and raise them with his mother's help. When he let impaired babies die, Haiselden always had the horrors of an institutional upbringing and existence in mind.

One thing the Baby Bollinger story proved was that Haiselden's views about euthanasia were not unique. The well-known American lawyer Clarence Darrow, future defense attorney during the Scopes "Monkey"

Trial of 1925, agreed wholeheartedly with Haiselden. When asked his opinion of the Baby Bollinger controversy, Darrow answered acerbically: "Chloroform unfit children. Show them the same mercy that is shown beasts that are no longer fit to live." Blind and deaf advocate Helen Keller added: "Our puny sentimentalism has caused us to forget that a human life is sacred only when it may be of some use to itself and to the world."[3]

The Baby Bollinger story stands out as an early example of what would happen with greater frequency as the twentieth century progressed. Later activists would attempt to promote euthanasia by going public about their unconventional views and actions. Militants hoped that openly defying conventional beliefs about euthanasia would stimulate debate and break down resistance to their cause. Haiselden knew that the dilemma faced by the baby's parents made for a heartrending human-interest story that would personalize the issue of euthanasia. Yet he also borrowed a strategy popularized by anarchists of his day: "propaganda of the deed," committing a bold act in the hopes of prodding others to take a radical position. As Haiselden explained, eugenics had "a million theories, each theory with ardent backers. . . . But it lacked drive." Haiselden concluded that "the times were crying for some one central deed—some decisive action that would draw together all these theories and beginnings of things into one definite crusade."[4]

In the early twentieth century, however, there was little public support for mercy killing of the disabled. Haiselden enjoyed the backing of people such as Clarence Darrow, Helen Keller, birth-control advocate William J. Robinson, sex-reformer Mary Ware Dennett, the editorial board of the *New Republic*, novelist Jack London, and Eugene V. Debs, the socialist candidate for the U.S. presidency in 1912. But there was little prospect of legislative, pro-euthanasia victories in any state or country, a sign that there was minimal popular backing for such a reform. Whatever headlines Haiselden had managed to capture in 1915, America's entry into World War I in 1917 bumped him off the front pages of the nation's newspapers. In 1919, he died forgotten in Cuba, conducting genetic experiments and still chasing his eugenic dreams.

In 1920, the Michigan Supreme Court ruled that helping someone to die was illegal. A Michigan man was convicted of first-degree murder and sentenced to life imprisonment for preparing the poisonous beverage that his dying and bedridden wife drank. The court upheld his conviction, ruling that it was irrelevant that she had wanted to end her life. Suicide, the justices declared, was not the issue. Helping someone to kill herself was.

Many American courts and medical practitioners, as well as the churches, were strongly opposed to euthanasia in the early twentieth century. Those opinions would have to change dramatically before euthanasia had any chance of being legalized.

RELIGIOUS REVIVAL IN AMERICA

The traumatic effects of World War I dealt a severe blow to the cultural influence of the churches in countries such as Germany and Britain. Yet, while the war may have weakened the religious faith of many Europeans, in the United States the situation was quite different. America's delayed entry into the conflict meant that its home front was spared many of the horrors experienced by continental Europeans, whose governments had mobilized entire nations to fight a bitter war that ultimately claimed the lives of 10 million combatants and civilians. In the 1920s, U.S. churchgoing actually began to rise, reversing its prewar decline. Between 1916 and 1926, church membership across the country increased a striking 31 percent. Evangelical Protestantism enjoyed a revival, strengthening the already robust opposition to euthanasia in America. The coming in 1920 of Prohibition, the outlawing of the sale and distribution of alcoholic beverages, reflected the power of American Protestants to shape policy-making. This moral reform campaign to stamp out the sin of drunkenness carried over into subsequent years, at least until Prohibition was repealed in 1933.

Meanwhile, countless U.S. Protestants were searching for a more emotionally satisfying form of religious experience. Pentecostal churches drew both black and white followers in the country's South and West. More and more Protestant Americans were tiring of the Social Gospel orientation of the mainstream denominations. Around the turn of the twentieth century, many mainline churches had deemphasized doctrine while promoting social reform activism. In the 1910s, a number of preachers, led by the celebrated evangelist Billy Sunday, sought to correct this trend. They began talking about "godless social service nonsense" and attacked the country's slack morals and "creampuff" religion. It was time, many Protestants agreed, to start reading the Bible again and concentrate on discovering the "road into the kingdom of God," in Sunday's words.[5]

Coinciding with this religious revival was the founding of the Fundamentalist movement, a reaction to the inroads of evolutionary theory and liberal modernist currents of thought into American culture. The term

"Fundamentalism" was taken from *The Fundamentals: A Testimony to the Truth*, a series of twelve volumes published between 1910 and 1915, underwritten by Milton and Lyman Stewart, two oil-industry magnates. Contributors included prominent scholars such as James Orr, B. B. Warfield, and W. J. Eerdman. *The Fundamentals* summed up the basic beliefs of conservative Christians and represented their new willingness to engage in public policy debates. Fundamentalists earnestly attempted to stem what they thought was the progress of secularism and the subjection of the Bible to the standards of verification used in the natural sciences. Fundamentalists instead stressed the unerring accuracy of the scriptures and belief in miracles such as Christ's resurrection and the virgin birth. In 1919, the movement organized as the World's Christian Fundamentals Association.

These currents in American religion emphasized the traditional Christian theology of suffering. In the words of the late nineteenth-century Anglo-American evangelist C. H. Spurgeon, "the greatest earthly blessing that God can give to any of us is health, with the exception of sickness. Sickness has frequently been of more use to the saints of God than health has." Spurgeon spoke from experience. Much of his later life was a litany of physical and emotional ailments. Yet, to him, his anguish was God's will. Even the suffering of loved ones had a divine meaning. Their "trials lead us to the realities of religion," Spurgeon concluded.[6]

Fundamentalists' fervor in drawing battle lines between themselves and the secular liberals they believed were their mortal enemies virtually guaranteed that sooner or later euthanasia would emerge as a contentious social issue. The more Darwinists, eugenicists, and social reformers supported euthanasia, the more these deeply religious Americans viewed a right to die as a threat to the traditional values on which the country was based. Drawn to theories about the end of the world and the second coming of Jesus Christ, American Evangelicals stressed preparing one's own soul for the moment of divine judgment. Nothing appeared to conflict with Christian teaching more than seeking a speedy and painless death in order to end the "blessing" of suffering.

POSTWAR EUROPEAN SECULARIZATION

While Evangelical Protestantism was reenergizing religion in postwar America, in Europe secularizing trends that predated the outbreak of World War I gathered momentum in the 1920s. In Britain and Germany, secularization helped to pave the way for the first signs of an organized euthanasia movement. World War I's horrific loss of life and the profound grief and mourning it caused shook the religious beliefs of countless Europeans. In Britain, the war dealt a powerful blow to organized religion.[7] It was difficult for clerics to maintain that life was sacred when it was spent so cheaply by politicians and generals. Between 1914 and 1918, over 700,000 British soldiers lost their lives. Each British soldier faced only a one in two chance of surviving without being killed, wounded, or imprisoned. Numerous members of the educated and affluent classes of Britain served in the war as officers, and actually suffered more casualties relative to other social classes. Many of these educated young men vividly and eloquently described their experiences fighting in the trenches. Their often cynical accounts of wartime service undermined faith in "God, King, and Country." When scepticism mounted about the churches' support for the national war effort, faith in traditional Christian teachings fell, such as the belief in the sanctity of human life, so critical to opponents of euthanasia. This was reflected during the war years in a drop in church membership relative to population size, a trend that persisted into the interwar period.

The war, an English euthanasia advocate proclaimed in 1931, "undoubtedly had a loosening and disintegrating effect upon old-established ideas, such as we have never seen before." Society's "whole outlook on life" had been altered.[8] Because so many men died without their bodies being recovered and buried according to traditional religious rituals, the war defied "hundreds of years of Christian history which had taught the importance of the good death and the hope of life eternal." In response, numerous British men and women sought their moral certainties outside familiar religious teachings. Widespread disenchantment with conventional value systems sparked rising interest in less orthodox forms of religious experience, including spiritualist methods of communicating with the dead. Frequently, a casualty of this process was the long-standing definition of a "good death." Postwar Britons found it increasingly difficult "to perceive positive meanings in the deaths of loved ones."[9] The ground had been laid for the emergence of the organized euthanasia movement in Great Britain. The same could be said for Germany.

BINDING AND HOCHE

In the face of World War I's appalling human losses, it was understandable that some individuals would more readily question customary understandings of life and death, including the advisability of euthanasia. The first signs of such questioning surfaced in Germany shortly after hostilities ended in 1918. Several leading German scientists, including members of Ernst Haeckel's Monist League, had advocated euthanasia in the early twentieth century. But debate over euthanasia took on a new urgency for defeated Germans in the wake of the battlefield carnage of World War I.

The severe deprivations suffered by the home front and the grim conditions of life on the war's front lines prompted some Germans after the armistice to draw invidious distinctions between the nation's dependent population and their countrymen who had sacrificed their lives in defense of their country. Many openly asked why the government should continue to feed, clothe, and house Germany's mentally and physically handicapped citizens. By the dawn of the twentieth century, Germany had 187 public asylums, and that did not count the German-language mental hospitals in Austria and Switzerland. It was not as if asylum inmates were spoiled. Wartime conditions triggered severe underfunding of German asylums, exacerbating overcrowding, affecting the supply of pharmaceuticals, and causing steep declines in inmate rations. Weight loss was extensive among patients, and their susceptibility to contagious disease rose dramatically. Over the course of the war, roughly 30 percent of the pre-1914 asylum population perished due to hunger, disease, neglect, or abuse. The situation remained grim into the 1920s, as governments continued to cut expenditures on asylums and actually closed some facilities. Nonetheless, between 1924 and 1929, the number of psychiatric patients leapt from 185,397 to more than 300,000. This abrupt swing in patient demographics convinced growing numbers of German scientists and physicians that individual patient needs took a backseat to the collective needs of society and future generations.

Against this backdrop of mounting frustration with the nation's dependent classes, two German professionals co-authored one of the most historically influential arguments in favor of legal euthanasia. *Permitting the Destruction of Unworthy Life*, by Professor of Law Karl Binding and Professor of Psychiatry Alfred Hoche, appeared in 1920 and provided an immediate boost to the on-again, off-again euthanasia debate in Germany.[10] From beginning to end, their short tract wove together themes that had already appeared in other printed justifications of euthanasia. First, *Permitting the Destruction of Unworthy Life* was suffused with the self-confidence often evident in the writings of Darwinists and eugenicists that they were helping to usher in a new, long-overdue age of "higher morality" based on the teachings of science. Binding and Hoche also borrowed heavily from the popular theory among German scientists that the individual counted for little in contrast to the community. Germany's postwar requirements, they argued, dictated that the nation's dependent population might have to be sacrificed to ensure that the state survived.

Binding and Hoche's publication was likewise important because it demonstrated how easily euthanasia could be justified philosophically once one accepted a right to kill oneself. Binding argued that there were no substantial differences among decriminalizing suicide, legalizing a terminally ill person's voluntary right to request a humane and painless death, permitting the mercy killing of unconscious dying individuals, and authorizing the killing of hospitalized defectives. This last category included persons, Binding contended, whose deaths would be welcomed by their caregivers, families, and themselves, if only their true wishes could be revealed. Certainly, the state had no interest in keeping them alive, Binding concluded. They were "the fearsome counter image of true humanity," and their existence was an insult to the many German soldiers ("the finest flower of humanity") who selflessly had sacrificed themselves on the battlefields of World War I. Their lives were "not just absolutely worthless, but even of negative value."

Hoche, for his part, echoed Binding's theory that the many inmates housed in Germany's private and state institutions were "constitutionally less valuable" than other citizens. But, as a doctor, he fittingly tended to emphasize more than Binding the necessity for an entirely new approach to medical ethics that would endorse the mercy killing of helpless mental patients. Hoche grimly called for the overthrow of the customary religious ideas about the sanctity of life and warned that the Hippocratic Oath was no longer relevant to the conditions of state medicine in the twentieth century. He enthusiastically hailed the coming of "a new age . . . operating with a higher morality," a time when "eliminating those who are completely mentally dead" would be viewed as "a permissible and useful act."

Permitting the Destruction of Unworthy Life did not have an immediate impact on German medical thinking. In the decade following its publication, some German physicians expressed their misgivings about Binding and Hoche and their attempt to codify a "secular ethics." They also warned about ranking human lives according to their economic usefulness to the state and attempting to determine which of their patients were living "ballast existences." But the march of events, including the coming of the Great Depression by the late 1920s, produced its own relentless logic. As unemployment soared, and tax revenues plunged, attention shifted as it had done in the early 1920s to the many handicapped patients housed in state asylums at public expense. Psychiatrists, frustrated with the never-ending chore of trying to treat chronically ill patients, increasingly voiced the opinion in the 1930s that the sick were a heavy drain on the nation's resources. By 1939, one asylum director announced, the only "serious" question was "whether to maintain this patient material under the most primitive conditions or to eradicate it."[11] This stark choice would radicalize growing numbers of physicians, social scientists, and policy-makers in the 1930s, and not only in Germany.

THE VOLUNTARY EUTHANASIA LEGALIZATION SOCIETY

As German sympathy for patients with disabilities was falling in the 1930s, activists in the Anglo-American world were starting to organize in the hopes of undermining opposition to euthanasia in their own countries. Before the decade was over, the first two pro-euthanasia organizations had been formed, the first in Great Britain and the second in the United States. Over the next thirty years, both groups remained severely underfunded, small in membership, and sharply limited in their influence on policy-making. But their appearance on the scene marked a significant breakthrough in the history of euthanasia. Before the 1930s, there had been little formal collaboration among euthanasia advocates. It was left to a handful of activists such as Harry Haiselden to try to advance the cause. With the founding of groups dedicated to convincing the public, government, and courts to legalize euthanasia, the euthanasia movement in the 1930s began to enjoy its first measure of desperately needed organizational unity and power.

At their origins, these euthanasia groups were anything but the products of mass, grassroots movements. They were due to the efforts of mostly elderly individuals from the opinion-making classes of society. In England, for example, it is likely that a euthanasia organization would never have been formed before World War II without the exertions of C. Killick Millard (1870–1952). In 1935, Millard, a retired public health physician from the Midlands city of Leicester, almost single-handedly founded the Voluntary Euthanasia Legalization Society (VELS). Millard was an excellent example of the kind of maverick that the euthanasia movement historically attracted. Throughout a career in preventive medicine that stretched back to 1901, Millard championed iconoclastic causes, including temperance, cremation, and birth control. Millard, like so many proponents of euthanasia on both sides of the Atlantic Ocean, was also an avid eugenicist. A member of England's Eugenics Society and Malthusian League, he keenly supported the sterilization of England's "C3" population, the "social problem group" that allegedly exhibited the highest rates of mental deficiency, fertility, pauperism, crime, ignorance, and physical disability. In fact, as Millard began planning the formation of England's first euthanasia organization between 1931 and 1935, he used his contacts with the country's eugenicists to boost the fledgling group's early membership. As a result, he was able to convince leading figures such as the sexologist Havelock Ellis, authors H. G. Wells and George Bernard Shaw, and scientist Julian Huxley—all converts to eugenics—to join the VELS. By 1938, fifty members of Britain's Eugenics Society had joined the VELS.

Alongside the fact that Millard came from Leicester, there was another pivotal reason the VELS was headquartered in that city. Leicester had a history of radical, nonconformist politics and religious dissent dating back to the nineteenth century. It was also a hotbed of eugenic and neo-Malthusian birth-control sentiment. It was fitting that the city's foremost public health official should have been someone like Millard, an individual temperamentally predisposed to challenge long-standing taboos regarding family privacy issues and reproductive politics.

The VELS did not wait long before launching a campaign to change England's laws to permit voluntary euthanasia. In 1936, Millard arranged to have a bill introduced in Britain's House of Lords that would make it legal for terminally ill adults to request medical aid in dying. The bill sparked some lively debate, but to no one's surprise, it was decisively defeated. Millard and the VELS had never expected the bill to pass. They considered it a victory that newspaper reporting of the debate over the bill provided them with some coveted publicity.

When some VELS members expressed immoderate views in public, however, the group's leadership was much less thrilled. Try as they might to depict the VELS as solely interested in voluntary euthanasia, Millard and the group's board found it difficult to silence members who wanted to legalize involuntary euthanasia. In 1932, one future VELS member endorsed "the lethal chamber . . . for infants with gross defects" if their parents were willing to provide permission. Another British euthanasia advocate similarly favored euthanasia for "children suffering hopeless and terrible lives," if necessary without the knowledge of the parents. In his eyes, these children were "a prey on normal people" and ought to be put to death humanely.[12]

One outspoken euthanasia supporter was Ernest W. Barnes, the Anglican bishop of Birmingham, who urged the eugenic extermination of the feebleminded and other defectives. They were "doomed from birth to a subhuman existence," Barnes argued, and only society's "false humanitarianism" kept them alive. Such opinions may have resonated with a distinct minority in favor of euthanasia, but they also reinforced what critics of the VELS contended: that many of Millard's VELS colleagues were not content to limit euthanasia to only consenting, informed, and dying adults. The small but vocal Roman Catholic press in Britain again and again attacked Millard and VELS. Letitia Fairfield, a Catholic and senior medical officer for the London County Council (and sister of author Rebecca West), warned that if the VELS bill ever passed, the mentally handicapped would be "murdered" and homes for the aged poor would become "slaughter-houses." As the *Catholic Herald* put it in 1934, "the people who advocate euthanasia always advocate it for somebody else."[13]

THE EUTHANASIA SOCIETY OF AMERICA

The Euthanasia Society of America (ESA), founded in 1938 and headquartered in New York City, was the brainchild of two people, the wealthy New Yorker Ann Mitchell and the ex-Unitarian minister Charles Potter. Mitchell was a highly eccentric and abrasive individual whose emotional problems led to a stay in a U.S. psychiatric hospital (1934–1936) and likely contributed to her death in 1942 when she threw herself out the window of a Miami hotel. Her difficulties living with psychosis convinced her that euthanasia was a relief for the many other Americans suffering from mental illness, whether they requested it or not. She believed that mental diseases were chiefly due to heredity, and this naturally made her sympathetic to eugenics. In a lively and sometimes hair-raising correspondence with Millard, she talked of the seeming necessity of breeding human beings "as carefully as we do animals." She welcomed the coming of World War II because, she claimed, it gave both the United States and Britain an opportunity to do some serious "biological house cleaning." Mitchell's frank views were shared by few members of the ESA, but she was indulged because her financial contributions to the cause were sorely needed.[14]

Convinced of the need to legalize voluntary and involuntary euthanasia, Mitchell was thrilled in 1936 when she learned that both had been ardently defended by clergyman Charles Potter (1885–1962). Potter, born in Marlboro, Massachusetts, and ordained a Baptist minister in 1908, made headlines across the country for backing birth control, the equality of women, the League of Nations, and the abolition of capital punishment. In 1913, he joined the Unitarian ministry, but even that church proved to be too doctrinaire for his tastes. By the early 1930s, Potter had embraced humanism, founding the First Humanist Society of New York in 1929. Other members of the First Humanist Society included Columbia University philosopher John Dewey, scientists Albert Einstein and Julian Huxley, and author Thomas Mann. By 1937, the society and its branch organizations in England, France, Australia, and Russia numbered some 15,000 members. The First Humanist Society, Potter boasted, had no creed, clergy, or prayer.

Potter's efforts to promote humanism coincided with the signing of the 1933 Humanist Manifesto, a document chiefly scripted by two Unitarian ministers, Curtis W. Reese and John H. Dietrich, and signed by Potter and sixty Unitarian pastors. Their ideal was a universal church of humanity based on firm ethical commitments. Rejecting all notions of a transcendental God or an order of divine truth outside mankind, they believed in the sweeping improvability of human nature through scientifically based social engineering, and in whatever social causes freed individuals from traditional moral codes that limited human choice. These ideals led prominent Americans such as John Dewey to sign the manifesto. Dewey's emphasis on the development of the individual and learning through experience as keys to the growth of democracy dovetailed with the postulates of the Humanist Manifesto.[15]

To Potter, legalized euthanasia was an obvious humanist cause. He argued that permitting euthanasia emancipated humanity from mainstream value systems that forbade people from exercising their autonomy and developing their personalities to the fullest, even on their deathbed. People who freely chose euthanasia, Potter believed, were examples of true democracy in action. Euthanasia also curtailed human suffering, according to Potter. His experience as a "marryin' and buryin' parson" had exposed him to dying parishioners who pleaded with him to be put out of their misery. They deserved the liberty to receive medical help in dying, Potter concluded.

Despite his repeated invocations of individual freedom as a political goal, Potter, a supporter of involuntary eugenics and euthanasia, was no defender of laissez-faire personal choice. This was less of a contradiction than it appears. Although he and other Unitarians and humanists attacked traditional codes of conduct for blocking human freedom, they were not libertarians. If human beings were to be freed from long-standing moral and ethical beliefs, it was to enable them to make the right choices, not any choice whatsoever. Choice did not mean freedom to do what individuals pleased, but empowerment to do what a scientifically grounded humanism taught them to do.

Potter's deep faith in the liberating influence of science accounts for his belief in humanism and explains why he could condone coercive eugenics and euthanasia. In the 1920s, almost all American scientists were eugenicists to one degree or another, so Potter was convinced eugenics must be true. A Darwinist at heart, he also prized science for its capacity to undermine orthodox religious faith. His highly secularized form of religiosity led to an invitation to serve as adviser to Clarence Darrow's defense team at the 1925 Scopes "Monkey" Trial in Dayton, Tennessee. Later immortalized in the play and movie *Inherit the Wind*, the Scopes trial centered on a court challenge of Tennessee's law barring the teaching of evolutionary theory in the state's schoolrooms. Darrow and his client, John Scopes, a high school biology teacher, lost their case, and the state's law stayed on the books for another forty-two years. The trial has often been depicted as a showdown between objective science and irrational, intolerant religion. But things were not that simple. The textbook that Scopes used in his biology class included several favorable references to eugenics and the wisdom of human breeding.[16]

By the 1930s, Potter had become convinced that the next great crusade of his life would be convincing Americans that euthanasia should be permitted. Thus, he was happy to learn that Ann Mitchell was ready to bankroll a euthanasia organization, and in 1938 the Euthanasia Society of America became a reality. Just as the Voluntary Euthanasia Legalization Society enjoyed close ties to England's Eugenics Society, so there was remarkable overlap in membership between the ESA and the American Eugenics Society. A striking 73 percent of the ESA's founders were followers of eugenics. The eugenic orientation of the early ESA explained why, in Potter's words, the ESA initially backed "euthanasia for incurable idiots" as well as voluntary euthanasia. But the ESA under Potter's presidency quickly limited its mandate to promoting only elective euthanasia in state capitals. Like the VELS, the ESA realized only a voluntary euthanasia bill had any chance of being enacted. It drafted such a bill targeting only terminally ill adults but in 1939 could find no New York State legislators willing to introduce it into the state assembly. Potter remained undaunted, believing that once one state legislature enacted the ESA model bill, other states would follow suit and a broader bill would likely become a reality. "Our ultimate aim," Potter told Millard, was a bill legalizing the merciful killing of the incurably mentally handicapped. But first came persuading law-makers to pass voluntary euthanasia legislation.[17]

INEZ CELIA PHILBRICK

Another person who made impressive contributions to the early euthanasia movement was the flamboyant Nebraska physician Inez Celia Philbrick

(1866–1966), who led the unsuccessful campaign in that state to legalize medical mercy killing. Philbrick taught home economics at the University of Nebraska and, like Potter, supported world peace, birth control, women's suffrage, and an end to child labor. Philbrick's political iconoclasm was matched by her dissenting views about religion and organized medicine. A Unitarian, she also defended natural childbirth, midwifery, charity clinics, and socialized medicine. These viewpoints gradually earned her pariah status within her own profession, and she ultimately quit the American Medical Association. Yet her unconventional medical ideas never endangered her high reputation in her home state as a selfless physician who literally would brave fires and floods to deliver babies when other doctors were hard to find.

Philbrick, born in Bloomington, Wisconsin, stands out as a latter-day Annie Besant, who saw eugenics, euthanasia, and women's rights as kindred causes. She preached the Darwinist theory of sexual selection, which said women were "the guardians of the race." They were responsible for bringing children into the world, and thus the "sterilization of the unfit, which measure alone can save civilization from annihilation," was distinctly a women's issue. Philbrick's attitude toward euthanasia was similarly draconian; one of the purposes of euthanasia, she wrote, "is to remove from society living creatures so monstrous, so deficient, so hopelessly insane that continued existence has for them no satisfactions and entails a heavy burden on society."

A true pioneer in the history of the euthanasia movement, Philbrick had made a deathbed promise to a fellow physician to work for the legalization of euthanasia after the dying, pain-wracked woman had refused Philbrick's attempt to hasten her death, claiming she did not want Philbrick to face possible criminal prosecution. In 1937, Philbrick tried mightily but failed to get a euthanasia bill introduced into Nebraska's unicameral state legislature. Besides permitting voluntary euthanasia for incurably ill, mentally sound adults, her bill also contained a clause allowing "next of kin" to apply for euthanasia on behalf of "mental incompetents" and minors suffering from a fatal disability. When her bill failed in Nebraska, she moved to Ohio. Remembering the failed 1906 Ohio euthanasia bill, she had hopes that conditions in the Buckeye State would be more favorable for her lobbying efforts. They were not. In the words of the sole physician in Nebraska's legislature, Philbrick's campaign in favor of euthanasia was "twenty-five years too soon."[18]

Philbrick has unjustly been forgotten as an early crusader in the history of twentieth-century euthanasia. But her interpretation of euthanasia as a feminist and eugenic measure was not unique, and demonstrated that euthanasia was viewed by many reformers as an issue of particular concern for women.[19]

HIGH-PROFILE MERCY KILLINGS

The organized euthanasia movement was aided by unprecedented media coverage in the 1930s of the personal stories of people who either helped others to die or expressed their own wishes to die. According to *Time* magazine in 1939, mercy killings occurred in the United States at a rate of one a week, and the killers were seldom convicted. One person who told *Time* she wanted to die was Anna Becker, a former nurse from Buffalo, New York. Impoverished and in daily, excruciating pain because of severe injuries in a car crash two years earlier, Becker declared in a 1935 letter to the Erie County Medical Society: "I want to die. A competent physician could certainly kill me with less pain than I endure in an hour." But neither local physicians nor the American Medical Association would support her wishes and break the law.

American celebrities who committed high-profile suicides also helped to make euthanasia a frequent front-page story in the 1930s. George Eastman, founder of Eastman Kodak, fired a revolver into his heart one evening in 1932. Eastman took his own life in the midst of a lengthy illness and while depressed after watching a close friend endure a prolonged death. In a note he left behind, he wrote: "My work is done. Why Wait?" Numerous Americans, including the poet Carl Sandburg, expressed their admiration for Eastman's act, indicating that as the Great Depression unfolded, attitudes toward life and death were in flux.

An even more widely publicized suicide was that of the noted feminist Charlotte Perkins Gilman. Dying of cancer in 1935, Gilman penned a note that stated she "preferred chloroform to cancer." She then proceeded to kill herself in her Pasadena, California, home. But in an article published posthumously, she revealed that she thought euthanasia ought to apply to more than dying, consenting adults like herself. She asserted that euthanasia could be employed as "social surgery" for ridding civilization of its burdensome citizens. Despite these comments about the underprivileged and disadvantaged members of society, her defense of legal euthanasia was hailed by other American feminists, including Carrie Chapman Catt and Harriet Stanton Blatch.

The 1934 Brownhill case in England, involving a woman found guilty of murdering her son, gave euthanasia an added human-interest angle.

Sixty-two-year-old Mary Brownhill of Yorkshire had devoted her whole life to caring for her mentally handicapped son. When she learned she had to enter the hospital for a serious operation, she so feared for her son's safety that she drugged him and then killed him by injecting gas into him through a tube inserted in his mouth. The jury found her guilty of murder, the judge sentenced her to hang, but the home secretary pardoned her two days after she was sentenced. This case of mercy killing had nothing to do with voluntary euthanasia, but by personalizing the plight of parents such as Brownhill, it generated sympathy for her and others in the same position.

Several trials from this period demonstrated that courts would be willing to acquit people of murder in especially compelling cases. In 1939, Louis Greenfield of the Bronx killed his retarded seventeen-year-old son by placing two handkerchiefs soaked in chloroform over his mouth while he was sleeping. He was later acquitted of first-degree murder. In 1943, Massachusetts lawyer and Harvard graduate John Noxon was found guilty of electrocuting his six-month-old son, who had been born with Down syndrome. Noxon was sentenced to the electric chair. However, the governor of Massachusetts commuted Noxon's sentence to life imprisonment. Noxon served four and a half years of his sentence and was then released on parole. The jury had found him guilty because Noxon kept insisting that his son's death was an accident, despite evidence that a radio wire was found around the child's arm, and the child was on a metal tray and wearing wet diapers. On the other hand, Noxon suffered from polio, and sympathizers pointed out that he had a justifiable worry about trying to raise such a disabled child.

ESA and VELS spokespersons claimed the Noxon, Brownhill, and Greenfield cases indicated society was ready to approve euthanasia laws. What they really revealed was that defendants who killed the severely handicapped for genuinely merciful reasons were often treated leniently by juries and judges. If courts selectively refused to enforce laws against mercy killing or assisted suicide, it "reflected a pragmatic approach to the law, not a repudiation of it."[20]

INCREASING SUPPORT FOR EUTHANASIA

Public support in America and Britian for mercy killing was growing by the time World War II broke out, and some supporters of euthanasia openly challenged traditional teachings about the sacredness of life and the depravity of suicide. One Anglican minister questioned why Christianity and the state prohibited people from terminating their own lives with medical assistance when they knew they had a fatal and painful disease. Havelock Ellis put it more bluntly: the prohibition against merciful infanticide was simply "one of the unfortunate results of Christianity."[21] Many VELS and ESA members (and German scientists) believed that they were living in a new, enlightened age in which "orthodox morality," as C. Killick Millard called it, no longer applied to the changed conditions of life. Millard, Charles Potter, and others looked to science for the answers they claimed "orthodox morality" could not supply. Science supposedly furnished people with the means, knowledge, and duty to control human destiny, through policies such as eugenics and euthanasia. The worldwide economic and political crisis of the 1930s underlined the urgency of this radical yet seemingly necessary task.

Toleration of euthanasia was also beginning to grow in medical ranks in the 1930s. As before, the majority of doctors opposed anything resembling the legalization of assisted suicide or medical mercy killing. But signs from Britain and America suggested that the mainstreaming of euthanasia within the medical profession was not limited to the Third Reich. Some of the impetus for changing attitudes among physicians toward euthanasia derived from heightened awareness about cancer. In all industrialized countries, the proportion of elderly people was on the rise, and with more people reaching old age, the rate of cancer mortality jumped. It was no coincidence that several VELS members were involved in the Ministry of Health's Cancer Committee. It was also no coincidence that Clarence Cook Little, president of the American Society for the Control of Cancer, served as ESA president in the early 1940s. In the words of *Time* magazine in 1937, "more than any other disease, cancer has horrified the imagination of mankind. It kills slowly, painfully, and science does not yet know its causes or mechanism."[22] The mounting number of cancer deaths meant more and more people were enduring painful, protracted deaths, and Millard was not alone in thinking that this would stimulate demand for a right to die.

Millard and others who thought the dread of cancer would jump-start the euthanasia movement were actually thirty years ahead of their time. The 1930s may have looked like the best of times to start the euthanasia movement, but in other respects it was the worst of times. Even as the press helped to foster fears about cancer in the 1930s, it also fed the growing optimism that scientists would conquer the "dread disease" in future. The reputation of organized medicine was on the upswing, especially in the United States, where talk of a war on cancer was based on the perception that science and technology were triumphantly on the march. Great breakthroughs, including the discovery of antibiotics and the Salk vaccine for polio, were just around the corner. The image of the doctor as the scientific expert boldly and selflessly fighting diseases such as cancer was crystallizing at roughly the same time that the euthanasia movement was beginning. Confidence in the power of medical science would not begin to subside until the 1960s. In the meantime, doctors wanted to be known for what they could do to cure disease, not for giving in to illness and assisting the deaths of patients. As long as hope for a cure persisted, medical support for euthanasia as a remedy for cancer would remain weak.

Thus, as the 1930s drew to a close, Western society's attitudes toward euthanasia had not changed much. But they had changed. In the United States as in Europe, political, social, and economic developments of the 1930s constituted a crucible in which measures once thought objectionable became increasingly acceptable topics for discussion among people with influence over public policy. Toleration for programs that sought to extend state control over private, intimate matters such as reproduction and death was on the rise in certain professional circles, even though they remained minority positions.

American public opinion polls in 1937 and 1939 found support for some types of euthanasia. Of those polled, more actually favored death for deformed or mentally handicapped infants (45 percent) than voluntary euthanasia for terminally ill adults (37 percent). A British poll conducted just before World War II revealed similar trends in public opinion. When asked "Should those suffering from an incurable disease be allowed the option under proper medical safeguards of a voluntary death?" 62 percent were in favor, only 22 percent against, and 16 percent had no opinion. Since no earlier poll findings on euthanasia are extant, it is impossible to say how public attitudes toward euthanasia may have shifted in the twentieth century. But there is little doubt that public opinion was affected to some degree by the propaganda of euthanasia advocates in the 1930s.

These polling results thrilled euthanasia advocates such as Charles Potter and C. Killick Millard. Veterans of the campaigns to legalize eugenics and birth control, by the early 1940s they began to imagine that similar success for the euthanasia movement was imminent. But the next twenty years would demonstrate that these poll results were deceptive. Little did euthanasia proponents know that events occurring at roughly the same time in continental Europe would evoke widespread revulsion and set the euthanasia movement back an entire generation.

NOTES

1. H. Tristam Engelhardt Jr. and Edmund L. Erde, "Euthanasia in Texas: A Little Known Experiment," *Hospital Physician* 9 (1976): 30–31.

2. Martin S. Pernick, *The Black Stork: Eugenics and the Death of "Defective" Babies in American Medicine and Motion Pictures since 1915* (New York: Oxford University Press, 1996), 41.

3. Pernick, *The Black Stork*, 92.

4. Pernick, *The Black Stork*, 85.

5. James A. Morone, *Hellfire Nation: The Politics of Sin in American History* (New Haven: Yale University Press, 2002), 335.

6. Edward J. Larson and Darrel W. Amundsen, *A Different Death: Euthanasia and the Christian Tradition* (Downers Grove, Ill.: InterVarsity Press, 1998), 159–160.

7. Pat Jalland, *Death in the Victorian Family* (New York: Oxford University Press, 1996), 370.

8. N. D. A. Kemp, *"Merciful Release": The History of the British Euthanasia Movement* (Manchester: Manchester University Press, 2002), 90.

9. Jalland, *Death in the Victorian Family*, 380–381.

10. Richard Weikart, *From Darwin to Hitler: Evolutionary Ethics, Eugenics, and Racism in Germany* (New York: Palgrave Macmillan, 2004), 155–156.

11. Michael Burleigh, *Death and Deliverance: "Euthanasia" in Germany, 1900–1945* (Cambridge: Cambridge University Press, 1994), 89.

12. Ian Dowbiggin, "'A Prey on Normal People': C. Killick Millard and the Euthanasia Movement in Great Britain, 1930–1955," *Journal of Contemporary History* 36 (2001): 59–85.

13. Kemp, *"Merciful Release,"* 109.

14. Ian Dowbiggin, *A Merciful End: The Euthanasia Movement in Modern America* (New York: Oxford University Press, 2003), 50–54.

15. Paul K. Conkin, *American Originals: Homemade Varieties of Christianity* (Chapel Hill: University of North Carolina Press, 1997), 93.

16. Edward J. Larson, *Summer for the Gods: The Scopes Trial and America's Continuing Debate over Science and Religion* (New York: Basic, 1997).

17. Dowbiggin, *A Merciful End*, 50–61.

18. Valery Garrett, "The Last Civil Right? Euthanasia Policy and Politics in the United States, 1938–1991," Ph.D. dissertation, University of California at Santa Barbara, 1998, 14.

19. Dowbiggin, *A Merciful End*, 45–50.

20. Larson and Amundsen, *A Different Death*, 162.

21. Kemp, *"Merciful Release,"* 109.

22. James T. Patterson, *The Dread Disease: Cancer and Modern American Culture* (Cambridge, Mass.: Harvard University Press, 1987), 120–121.

5

IN GOD WE TRUST

The brief momentum the euthanasia movement enjoyed in the 1930s came to an abrupt halt within a decade. In 1939, the world plunged into war, and when news of Nazi atrocities began to filter out of central and eastern Europe, sympathy for euthanasia began a nosedive that lasted for two decades. To traditional opponents of euthanasia, chiefly the Roman Catholic Church, the Third Reich's experiment with euthanasia was proof that legalizing mercy killing was a serious mistake. Organized medicine tended to think the same way. Public opinion polls also registered diminished support for euthanasia in the 1950s. By the 1960s, the euthanasia movement had ground to a virtual standstill.

But not for long. If the campaign to enact euthanasia legislation was losing momentum by the 1960s, the broader topic of death and dying was receiving increased attention and would become a major interest for the balance of the twentieth century. Important technological innovations in the medical treatment of the terminally ill were beginning to spark a mounting debate over the issue of unnecessary and unwanted treatment. Support for a patient's right to reject futile treatment gave birth to the phrase "right to die." The right to die replaced euthanasia as the focus of debate. These and other changes indicated that the euthanasia movement's stalemate in the 1940s and 1950s was only a temporary lull in a long-term conflict over the value of human life.

NAZI MEDICAL MURDER

Under the conditions of total war between 1939 and 1945, the assault on traditional German medical ethics begun by Ernst Haeckel, Karl Binding, and Alfred Hoche became a horrific reality. Just before German military forces began ravaging central and eastern Europe in 1939, Adolf Hitler issued a secret order permitting Nazi doctors to put to death mentally and physically handicapped patients. Hitler's order unleashed a murderous rampage. By the end of World War II, some 200,000 of these men, women, and children had been killed, most by starvation, gassing, shooting, or lethal injection in asylums, hospitals, and clinics inside and outside Germany.

Nazi euthanasia was closely linked to the Holocaust, the systematic murder of roughly 6 million European Jews as well as Gypsies, Poles, and other groups considered "racially undesirable" by the Third Reich. Many of the doctors who worked with the Nazi euthanasia program had acquired knowledge about methods of gassing patients. When these doctors were reassigned to Poland, they put their technical knowledge into practice by helping to plan the mass extermination of Europe's Jews at notorious killing centers such as Belzec, Sobibor, and Treblinka.[1]

The full news about Nazi medical murder came out in 1946–1947 during the "doctor trials" that were part of the Nuremberg trials of Nazi war criminals. Twenty-three of the defendants in the doctor trials (all but three of them physicians) were charged with murdering sick or injured persons or conducting illicit human experiments. But trials of Nazi doctors for medical murder did not end with the Nuremberg proceedings. As late as 2004, an eighty-eight-year-old ear, nose, and throat specialist was charged with involvement in the starvation and overdosing of more than 150 mentally handicapped women and children at a euthanasia hospital near Jena, Germany.

The revelations of Nazi medical murder that surfaced during the Nuremberg trials were staggering enough. Equally riveting was the information about the historical origins of Nazi-era euthanasia. American psychiatrist Leo Alexander, a consultant to the U.S. Office of the Chief Counsel for War Crimes in Nuremberg, concluded from the postwar trials that Nazi medical murder had started "from small beginnings." Nazi euthanasia was not an accident of history, but a policy with a powerful ancestry dating back to Ernst Haeckel and late nineteenth-century eugenics and Social Darwinism. Once some German physicians and scientists began to accept that there were lives "not worthy to be lived," Alexander argued, it became easier to extend this concept beyond the disabled and chronically ill to "the socially unproductive, the ideologically unwanted, the racially unwanted, and finally all non-Germans."[2]

Indeed, pro-euthanasia discourse inside and outside organized German medicine had been building gradually up to 1933, when Hitler's Nazi party came to power. By the time Hitler had emerged on Germany's political scene in the 1920s, many believed that society's interests were more important than the value of single individuals. Leading Germans increasingly measured the value of human lives according to standards such as happiness, pleasure, usefulness, or economic productivity. From there it was a small step to thinking that the benefits of a quick and painless death should be extended to persons whose lives failed to meet these standards, even if they were incapable of giving their permission. Under the conditions of total war, when Germans were expected to make the ultimate sacrifice for the nation, it was decidedly difficult to resist the thinking that underlay euthanasia. Questioning such survivalist reasoning was tantamount to treason.

Hitler propounded the view that extreme circumstances demand extreme measures. His Social Darwinist perspective convinced him that, even in peacetime, Germany was on a war footing. Throughout the interwar period, he declared in speeches that Germany's "modern sentimental humanitarianism" meant society maintained the "weak at the expense of the healthy." As Hitler wrote in his 1925 autobiography *Mein Kampf* ("My Struggle"), the blueprint of the Nazi movement, the nation had to make "a new and ruthless choice according to strength and health." In an unpublished 1928 manuscript, Hitler revealed how Darwinism, eugenics, and infanticide intersected in his way of thinking: "While nature only allows the few most healthy and resistant out of a large number of living organisms to survive in the struggle for life, people restrict the number of births and then try to keep alive what has been born, without consideration of its real value and its inner merit. Humaneness is therefore only the slave of weakness and thereby in truth the most cruel destroyer of human existence."[3] Thus, when begged in 1938 by a German family named Knauer to permit physicians to kill their blind and deformed infant son, Hitler decided the time was ripe to launch a euthanasia program.

However, there were two chief problems. The first was his reluctance to enact a formal law legalizing the murder of handicapped adults and children. Even after years of Nazi propaganda and indoctrination, Hitler was understandably worried about the backlash from German Christians if he openly advocated euthanasia. Hitler was already planning for war and did not want to do anything that might jeopardize national morale and unity. The second problem was that physicians would never comply with such a program for fear of prosecution. So Hitler signed a document on his personal stationery ordering a group of Nazi officials to set up a covert bureaucracy intended to register, select, and murder a target group of handicapped people that included schizophrenics, epileptics, disabled babies, and other long-stay hospital patients. The program became known as "Aktion T-4," after the address of its headquarters in a Berlin suburb.

Just as Hitler feared, news about Aktion T-4 leaked out, and in 1941 he ran into opposition from a few Protestant and Roman Catholic clergy in Germany. One, Clemens August Graf von Galen, the Catholic bishop of Munster, denounced the T-4 operation from his pulpit. Later, the Royal Air Force leafleted copies of his sermon over Germany. Hitler and the Nazi leadership thought of liquidating Galen but decided to postpone the bishop's punishment until after the war. In the meantime, they directed that the entire operation become decentralized, more covert, and more difficult to monitor. Many of Aktion T-4's doctors fanned out into the death camps, where they collaborated in the selection of "sick" inmates for extermination. The medical killers remained busy in asylums, clinics, and concentration camps until the end of World War II.

MILLARD, MITCHELL, AND NAZI EUTHANASIA

Even before the full extent of Nazi medical murder surfaced at the Nuremberg doctor trials of 1946–1947, news of killings of psychiatric patients and disabled infants had trickled out of eastern Europe. As early as the winter of 1939–1940, the Vatican and journalists such as William Shirer were reporting that entire Polish asylums were being emptied by mass shootings of patients. At first, euthanasia advocates in America and Britain hoped the stories would quickly fade from the news. But when they did not, the executive boards of the ESA and VELS scrambled to adjust their programs so they would not be associated with Nazi involuntary euthanasia. In the midst of World War II, the ESA abruptly shelved its plans to promote a state bill that would have permitted the mercy killing of patients such as the Knauer family's blind and deformed infant son. The ESA, like the VELS, decided that public pronouncements in favor of involuntary euthanasia should cease, at least until the war ended and supposedly cooler heads prevailed. In the short term, the two groups resolved to seek the legalization of only voluntary euthanasia.

Most ESA and VELS members took to heart the advice to refrain from voicing support for involuntary euthanasia to the press. But some members, in their communications with one another, showed that they had not changed their minds. For example, before her death in 1942, Ann Mitchell, financial mainstay of the ESA, found an outlet for her neo-Nazi views in her wartime letters to C. Killick Millard of the VELS. While wishing that the mental patients dispatched by Nazi doctors could have been murdered less painfully, she still hoped that the war would "last a long time." In her opinion, the longer the war, the more favorable the conditions for advocating "euthanasia as a war measure, including euthanasia for the insane, feeble-minded monstrosities, thus saving food, medicine, housing, medical care and nursing to help to win the war." Underlining her deep sympathy for Nazi Germany's goals, if not its exact methods, Mitchell told Millard that it was in the interests of the wartime Allies that they follow the Third Reich's euthanasia example.

Millard was acutely sensitive about the potential for bad public relations if VELS members advocated euthanasia for people with disabilities. But, like Mitchell, Millard saw a distinct silver lining when war broke out in 1939. In his 1940 report to the VELS, Millard asserted that the current war, like World War I, would modify "old standards" about biomedical ethics and make "new ideas" about the value of human life more palatable.[4] The "new idea" he cherished the most was the acceptance of an individual right to a speedy and painless death to relieve unremitting pain.

After the war, Millard's stance on euthanasia surfaced in a series of events that, if they had been exposed to public scrutiny at the time, would have done serious damage to the VELS. In June 1950, Millard received a letter from an imprisoned Austrian former Waffen Schutzstaffeln (SS) doctor named Siegbert Ramsauer. In 1947, a British military tribunal had found Ramsauer guilty on two counts of involuntary euthanasia performed on POWs at the Loibl Pass work camp, affiliated with the infamous Mauthausen concentration camp near Linz, Austria. Ramsauer did not ask Millard for help in reopening his case (he never denied his actions) but simply requested that Millard help him receive clemency from the British king so he could rejoin his family in Austria.

In the words of the prosecuting attorney in 1947, Ramsauer had joined the SS because "he firmly believed and still believes in the Nazi doctrines and would be an ideal member for any Nazi underground movement." There was nothing in Ramsauer's career that would have belied such an interpretation. From 1935 to 1940, Ramsauer had studied medicine at the University of Vienna medical school. In 1938, shortly after the Nazi takeover of Austria, 153 of the 197 members of Vienna's faculty of medicine were fired, most because of Jewish origins or having married Jews. Under the leadership of the outspoken Nazi Edouard Pernkopf, the author of what later became a classic anatomy text, Vienna's curriculum was reconstructed to conform to Nazi ideology. Students received a heavy indoctrination in eugenics, euthanasia, and racial hygiene. They were taught that the health of the individual was subordinate to the overall fitness and fertility of the nation. First and foremost, the physician was to be the servant of the Führer and his people, not individual patients.

Ramsauer's medical training at Vienna prepared him to join the SS in July 1940. After stints at Mauthausen and the Dachau concentration camp, in 1943 Ramsauer was appointed head physician at the Loibl work camp. Besides being charged with ill-treatment and neglect of prisoners and the withholding of medicine from laborers, he was held responsible for ordering the killing of at least two severely injured workers. At his trial in 1947, Ramsauer claimed he was only following orders. Yet Ramsauer was not a victim of bad luck, an unfortunate person caught in the wrong place at the wrong time. It was no accident that SS doctors like Ramsauer performed so many atrocities in World War II, including medical murder. Death meant something different to them than it did to ordinary doctors, who were respected for their healing powers. SS doctors were recognized as wielding the power of death. Patients were very much at the mercy of SS doctors, many of whom took the symbolism of death surrounding the SS very seriously. Medical murder, painless or otherwise, was just another form of health care to SS doctors.

As Millard wrote after receiving Ramsauer's letter, "I cannot help feeling very sorry for Dr. Ramsauer." Nonetheless, no one in the British War Office or Foreign Office listened to Millard's pleas. Ramsauer remained in prison until 1954, when the Foreign Office finally recommended his release.[5] Clearly, Ramsauer was a second-rank Nazi criminal whose actions paled in comparison with the other German physicians convicted at Nuremberg. Still, Millard's willingness to help Ramsauer was unsettling. The memory of the Nazi doctors' trial at Nuremberg was fresh in the public mind. Millard also knew that he was sympathizing with a convicted war criminal. But from Millard's perspective, Ramsauer's pro–euthanasia views trumped everything else. He felt a kinship for anyone who shared his support for euthanasia, even a war criminal. Millard was certainly no Nazi, nor was Ann Mitchell. Yet their views about euthanasia shared some disturbing similarities with the opinions of German doctors who committed crimes against humanity under the Nazi regime.

THE EUTHANASIA MOVEMENT STALLS

News of Millard's efforts on Ramsauer's behalf never saw the light of day. But the fortunes of the euthanasia movement were shaky enough in the late

1940s and throughout the 1950s. In 1950, the VELS tried for the second time for legislative success. Lord Chorley, acting on behalf of the VELS, proposed in the British House of Lords that the government accept the principle of voluntary euthanasia, but the result was as discouraging as it was in 1936. Chorley, sensing that the opposition was overwhelming, withdrew his motion before a vote was taken. One opponent, the Archbishop of York, declared: "If once we begin to allow legislation of this kind we put our feet on a very slippery slope." Chorley fed the fears that the euthanasia movement had a hidden agenda when he admitted that "children who come into the world deaf, dumb, and crippled . . . have a much better case than [the adults] for whom the Bill provides."[6]

The World Medical Association and the British Medical Association issued crystal-clear condemnations of euthanasia in 1950. Two years later, Millard died, a serious setback to the VELS, roughly coinciding with the death or retirements of several other leading VELS members. By then, the VELS had learned yet another tough lesson in the politics of euthanasia advocacy. It was hard sustaining momentum and continuity in the movement when the majority of people who gravitated to the cause in the first place were elderly. Young people, less concerned about their own mortality, were difficult to attract to the movement and mobilize as activists. This was reflected in the VELS membership, which showed only 226 paying members in 1955, roughly twenty years after the group had been formed.

As stymied as the British euthanasia movement was during the early stages of the Cold War, in America the movement fared even worse. Not that there were no high points. The trial of the physician Hermann Sander in 1949–1950 gripped the imagination of the nation and the world unlike any euthanasia-related news since the story of pro-euthanasia surgeon Harry Haiselden. Sander was a New Hampshire general practitioner who was charged with killing a fifty-nine-year-old cancer patient by injecting air into her arm as she lay dying in a hospital bed and wracked with severe pain. After a fourteen-day trial in early 1950 in the small town of Candia, New Hampshire, the jury ruled that Sander's actions had not killed the patient, and he was acquitted.

The verdict was hailed by his many supporters, who deeply admired Sander's compassion as a family doctor. But he received little sympathy from his colleagues in organized medicine. Local medical societies stripped him of his license to practice and his hospital privileges. Religious reaction was more mixed. The Vatican newspaper *Osservatore Romano* stated that mercy killing "injects the poison of atheism into the veins of society." Indeed, few religious spokespersons outright approved of Sander's actions. However,

many sympathized with Sander, including the distinguished Protestant theologian Reinhold Niebuhr. The budding evangelist Billy Graham insisted that
the taking of life was murder under any circumstances, but he still thought
Sander was a "good man. Many of our sympathies are with him. . . . But he
was misdirected and misled in what he did."[7]

Perhaps the most startling aspect of the Sander trial was the huge
crowd of over 150 reporters and photographers who descended on tiny
Candia. They came from across the country and from as far away as London, England, and they swamped switchboard operators and Western Union
clerks with roughly 200,000 words a day. John O'Hara and Fanny Hurst
were just two of the many prominent writers who commented in print on
Sander's trial. Hurst, an ESA member, was predictably sympathetic to
Sander. "Not Since Scopes?" asked *Time* magazine rhetorically, hinting that
no trial had seen so much media coverage or been so important since the
1925 Scopes Trial over the teaching of evolution in Tennessee public
schools.[8]

However, once the trial was over, the Sander story vanished from the
newspapers, and the euthanasia issue rapidly faded from public consciousness. ESA activists, who had hailed the Sander trial as a watershed in the history of their movement, soon learned that the public had a very short attention span. Not until the Karen Ann Quinlan story of 1974–1976 would
press coverage of euthanasia leave such a deep imprint on public opinion.
Hermann Sander soon became a footnote to history. By contrast, Karen
Ann Quinlan became an internationally famous name and face.

Gallup polls in the postwar period confirmed that, despite all the sympathy for Hermann Sander, public opinion did not favor legal euthanasia. In
1950, one poll asked Americans: "When a person has a disease that cannot
be cured, do you think doctors should be allowed by law to end the patient's
life by some painless means if the patient and his family request it?" In 1939,
46 percent of those polled had answered yes. In 1950, only 36 percent
replied yes. The alarming (and fairly accurate) conclusion euthanasia proponents drew was that support for euthanasia was slipping, despite all their
efforts at public education.

On the legislative front, the U.S. euthanasia movement faced yet more
disappointment. Hopes for a victory in New York State evaporated in the
early 1950s, partially because of failed efforts to enlist medical support for a
voluntary euthanasia bill in the Empire State. A similar effort in Connecticut in 1959 went down to defeat. Initially, things went well for the ESA in
New York. In the late 1940s, the group was able to obtain hundreds of
physicians' signatures to a petition urging New York State legislators to vote

for a bill permitting terminally ill patients over the age of twenty-one to ask their doctors to end their lives painlessly. But state and national medical societies across the United States, including the American Medical Association (AMA), roundly condemned legalized euthanasia. Then, in the face of militant opposition from medical groups, many of the doctors who signed the ESA petition backed down and publicly denounced the organization. The experience proved to the ESA once again that, while some doctors believed euthanasia was appropriate in some instances, organized medicine was nowhere near ready to approve of mercy killing.

The opposition of organized medicine to euthanasia stemmed from more than physicians' refusal to identify themselves with anything that suggested they could not cure their patients. Medical opposition to euthanasia also derived from the inherently conservative nature of the profession during the first half of the twentieth century, especially in the United States. For much of this period, for example, the AMA fought tooth and nail against any forms of national health insurance, denouncing them as creeping communism. Euthanasia, whose opponents sometimes equated it with Nazism or Soviet communism, ended up being tarred with the same brush as socialized medicine. When a national health program became a possibility in 1948 after Harry Truman was elected president, the AMA launched a massive public relations campaign to convince the American people that socialized medicine was a bad idea. Medical research, a member of Congress exclaimed in the 1950s, was "the best kind of health insurance." An American doctor remarked that "the only genuine medical insurance for this country lies in making the benefits of science available to all practitioners and to all patients."[9]

This pro-science bravado of American culture during the Cold War played a critical role in the debate over euthanasia. With politicians openly celebrating the prospect of medical science conquering disease, and with the strong cultural aversion to radical policy experiments, there could be little hope that widespread support for euthanasia was imminent.

RELIGIOUS OPPOSITION

By the early 1950s, the ESA knew it could count on the support of many Unitarian ministers. The Unitarian-Universalist Association affirmed the right to die in 1988, but even before that date, its clergy tended to sympathize with euthanasia. In 1948, the ESA sponsored a public statement declaring euthanasia ethical. Of the fifty clergy who signed, twenty were pastors at Unitarian or Universalist churches. Celebrating the Social Gospel, abandoning all creeds, opposing all forms of fatalism, encouraging individuals to create their own value systems, and generally subscribing to every liberal cause, Unitarians were viscerally predisposed to support voluntary euthanasia.

Similar support from America's other churches, however, was not forthcoming. Charles Potter, founder of the First Humanist Society, told Millard in 1938 that the only "serious" opposition to the ESA came from the Roman Catholics and "the orthodox fundamentalist groups," but religious resistance to euthanasia was much broader than that. American Judaism refused to countenance either mercy killing or assisted suicide, and many rabbis emphatically spoke out against euthanasia. The president of the Lutheran Church Missouri Synod condemned euthanasia, as did U.S. Presbyterians and Methodists. They were joined by the American Council of Christian Churches, with its million and a half members, and the General Convention of the Protestant Episcopal Church.

Nonetheless, the most formidable foe of euthanasia continued to be the Roman Catholic Church. By the 1950s, Catholicism wielded sweeping political and cultural clout in the United States. Movie and television executives were so fearful of Catholic condemnation that they eliminated scenes of sex and violence from their shows. When the Catholic Church was depicted in films, such as *Going My Way* and *The Bells of St. Mary's*, it was in uniformly positive fashion. Even popular television comedians, such as Milton Berle, had to take a programming backseat to Catholic Bishop Fulton J. Sheen's *Life Is Worth Living* program. In the 1950s, no U.S. church enjoyed more power than the Roman Catholic Church.

American Catholicism's heyday coincided with the country's robust religiosity of the 1950s. Congress deferred to this revival of religious sentiment by adding the words "under God" to the Pledge of Allegiance and the phrase "in God we trust" to all U. S. currency. President Dwight D. Eisenhower regularly opened cabinet meetings with a prayer. This "new piety" struck some observers as bland and theologically challenged, but there was no discounting how, as a new "civic religion," it undermined whatever broad societal trends had been working in the euthanasia movement's favor since the Depression.[10]

Catholic might was built on its demographic success. Catholicism's share of the national population grew from 19 percent to 23 percent between 1930 and 1960. Catholics also tended to cluster in big cities such as New York, Chicago, Boston, and Philadelphia, giving the church impressive political strength. Brooklyn held a million Catholics in 1930. Catholic electoral strength meant that, when the ESA attempted to organize a campaign to introduce voluntary euthanasia legislation in New York State in the late 1940s, no member of the state assembly would risk political suicide backing such an endeavor. The power of the church at the ballot box ensured that the Catholic position on sensitive social issues tended to become national and state policy. Thanks to the church's similar influence on the nation's popular culture, its doctrines of ethical and moral conduct reached well beyond the faithful to affect non-Catholics as well.

In the late 1940s, the power of the Roman Catholic Church in the United States triggered a bitter culture war between the church and American liberals, the opening act in the divisive conflict of the late twentieth century over abortion. In the years leading up to the Great Depression of the 1930s, American liberals actually had few profound disagreements with the Catholic Church. Common ground between liberals and Catholics was frequently found in their shared admiration for state economic planning and a more equitable distribution of the nation's wealth. Many U.S. liberals were sincerely dismayed over the anti-Catholic prejudice that helped to fuel the rise of the Ku Klux Klan in the 1920s and scuttled Democratic Party candidate Al Smith's 1928 campaign for the presidency.

However, in the 1930s, more and more U.S. liberals grew concerned about Catholic support for political causes they deemed dangerous. For example, many Catholics, among them radio celebrity Father Charles E. Coughlin, openly sympathized with dictators such as Italy's Benito Mussolini and Spain's Francisco Franco. Senator Joseph McCarthy's overwrought search for communists in the early 1950s, a campaign backed by many U.S. Catholics, convinced liberals that their misgivings about Catholic intentions had been vindicated.

To an increasing number of American liberals, including John Dewey, Lewis Mumford, Horace Kallen, and the editorial board of the *New Republic*, the Roman Catholic Church was an outdated relic of medieval authoritarianism surviving into the twentieth century. Many went further and insisted its presence constituted a worrisome threat to American democracy, equal to the brainwashing power of Soviet communism. Because of the millions of American children enrolled in Catholic parochial schools, liberals worried that church teachings would harm national unity, delay the progress of science and technology, and jeopardize the personal autonomy of countless future U.S. citizens. To Dewey, the Catholic Church over the centuries had been engaged in a disturbing and "systematic stultification of the human mind and human personality." No wonder he believed that its views were incompatible with the democratic values of the United States.

Armed with these suspicions, American liberals staged a concerted counter-attack against the church's influence. They flocked to organizations such as the American Civil Liberties Union (ACLU) and Protestants and Other Americans United for the Separation of Church and State (POAU). Liberals aggressively lobbied government and the courts to erect a "wall of separation" between public institutions (such as schools) and organized religion. In 1947, the leader of the American Unitarian Association, in a thinly veiled jab at Catholicism, called for a Christianity "free of all autocratic ecclesiastical control over the mind and conscience of its individual members."[11] By this time, liberals were not content merely to protect non-Catholics from the church's influence. They wanted to liberate Catholics from their own church's hierarchy and doctrines.

PAUL BLANSHARD

Opponents of Catholic Church doctrine often berated the church for its teaching on sex and reproduction. Catholicism taught that conjugal acts were solely for the begetting of children, and only abstinence was permissible as a method of contraception. But Catholic doctrine on euthanasia also infuriated many liberals. And no one wished to free Americans from these church doctrines as desperately as Paul Blanshard, author of the 1949 runaway best-seller *American Freedom and Catholic Power*. Indeed, to many liberals in the United States such as Blanshard, the struggle to decriminalize euthanasia was an important pillar of the entire crusade to emancipate Americans from an authoritarian church. Whether it was euthanasia or birth control, the church seemingly could not desist from interfering in the private lives of democratic citizens, and to Blanshard and other liberals, it had to be stopped.

Blanshard's *American Freedom and Catholic Power* was first serialized in the *Nation*, a bastion of left-liberal opinion. His book was a blistering attack on the church hierarchy's influence over politics, education, the labor movement, and the arts. Blanshard, a trustee of the Ethical Culture Society and follower of John Dewey, believed that the church was an obstacle to progress in a century marked by astounding advances in science, technology, and the economy. He particularly castigated the church for its teachings on marriage, divorce, birth control, and sex education. These doctrines, Blanshard alleged, prevented Americans from developing the emotional and cognitive skills to adapt to the rapid social, political, and economic changes of the twentieth century.

Blanshard's book also contained strong approval of euthanasia and eugenic sterilization. In his day, many scientists were turning away from eugenics, troubled by its association with Nazism and the outlandish statements by some of its proponents. But that did not bother Blanshard. He vigorously denounced the Catholic Church for frustrating attempts to enact state sterilization laws across the country. "Meanwhile," he wrote, "the feeble-minded who are at large in our population produce future Americans at a much faster rate than our normal citizens." Operating on the notion that the enemy of my enemy must be my friend, he also lauded the ESA for its efforts to legalize euthanasia in the face of stiff Catholic opposition. Blanshard likewise endorsed the ESA because it claimed to support an individual's right to request medical aid in dying, which he believed was a genuine exercise of personal freedom.[12] Blanshard may have insisted all along that he was only upholding the individual's right to choose, but he turned a blind eye toward the considerable sentiment within the ESA for involuntary euthanasia. Similarly, he never addressed how coercive state sterilization laws were consistent with a nation founded on the principle of personal autonomy.

CATHOLIC BIOETHICS

Blanshard's stalwart backing of euthanasia and eugenic sterilization did not prevent noted liberals such as John Dewey and Albert Einstein from hailing his book as a weapon in the struggle against the Catholic Church's sway over America's value systems. Indeed, *American Freedom and Catholic Power* was a passionate attempt to counter the success of Catholic theologians who by the mid-twentieth century had constructed a sophisticated body of writings telling nurses, doctors, and patients what to do in complex medical situations. In 1947, the first Catholic code of medical ethics was drafted, shaping clinical and administrative decisions in hundreds of Catholic hospitals in the United States and Canada. To liberal theologians who wanted to counter Catholic influence over birth control, eugenics, and euthanasia policy-making, the church's success in these areas was dismaying. As one critic of Catholic power grudgingly noted in 1954, "Catholic literature on the morals of medical care is both extensive and painstaking in its technical detail, while Protestant and Jewish literature is practically non-existent." A secular body of writings on the same topic was conspicuously missing.[13] That would change in the 1960s with the emergence of the field of biomedical ethics, and in particular the founding of the Hastings Center in 1970, the leading twentieth-century think-tank in medical ethics. But, in the meantime, Catholic moral theologians such as John C. Ford and John A. Ryan tended to dominate the national debate over the rules and norms of medical conduct.

Father John A. Ryan, the pivotal American figure in early twentieth-century Catholic social theory, had predicted repeatedly that society's innocent and vulnerable groups would suffer if governments deviated from the church's stance on the sanctity of life. For centuries, the Catholic Church had taught that someone's suffering a painful death was not a justification for permitting mercy killing. "No one suffers save through the will of God," contended a twentieth-century American priest; "through suffering a man can beautify his character, atone for his sins, [and] take a special part in the sublime work of the Redemption."[14] Throughout the 1930s, Catholic spokespersons, following Pope Pius XI's 1930 encyclical *Casti Connubii*, time and again pointed to eugenics and euthanasia as examples of what ignoring church teaching would lead to.

After World War II, Father John C. Ford, another highly influential Catholic ethicist, explained that once people started believing humans were the masters of their lives, not God, and that humans had a right not to suffer, it would not be long before innocent life would be endangered. Joseph Sullivan, the American author of *Catholic Teaching on the Subject of Euthanasia* (1947), the first book on that particular subject, concurred that "once the American people depart so far from Christian tradition as to allow an innocent person to be put to death because he is a monstrosity or wills euthanasia, it is difficult to predict how much further this abuse of human life will go."[15] This slippery-slope argument exerted a profound influence over post-1945 medical ethics. Although not a Catholic himself, psychiatrist Leo Alexander said much the same thing with his theory that Nazi medical murder had started with "small beginnings."

GLANVILLE WILLIAMS AND JOSEPH FLETCHER

To those opposed to the Catholic Church's influence, Catholic leadership in the field of medical ethics was intolerable, sparking a spirited reaction that began in the 1950s on both sides of the Atlantic Ocean and gathered momentum over the next few decades. The University of London's Glanville Williams and former Episcopal clergyman Joseph Fletcher stand out as pioneering bioethicists opposed to church doctrine. Neither came to the field of medical ethics as disinterested scholars with no preconceived ideas. In their eagerness to overturn church teachings, however, they both fell prey to the same enthusiasm for involuntary euthanasia and eugenics as Blanshard's.

Williams, a distinguished criminal lawyer and admirer of utilitarian principles, was a supporter of abortion rights, eugenic sterilization, and reform of laws directed against homosexuality. He was already a VELS member when in 1958 he published *The Sanctity of Life and the Criminal Law*, in which he took direct aim at the "double effect" doctrine of the Catholic Church. This doctrine stated that as long as the patient had given permission and the physician was only trying to alleviate pain, there was no sin involved in a doctor administering narcotics even if it brought about an earlier death. As recently as February 1957, Pope Pius XII had reaffirmed this theory. Yet Williams, like Samuel D. Williams in the late nineteenth century, thought it was plain nonsense. What did it matter, he asked, when the effect was the same whether the aim was to minimize pain or actually hasten death?

According to Glanville Williams, voluntary euthanasia was perfectly justifiable, but so was involuntary euthanasia of severely handicapped infants. Williams subscribed to ideas reminiscent of Binding and Hoche when he argued that the legality of euthanasia chiefly depended on the future happiness and social usefulness of individuals. If a person's quality of life appeared compromised by illness or disability, then mercy killing was a virtuous act, as was withholding treatment that would prolong life. In fact, Williams added, the number of "degenerate" children was increasing thanks to modern medicine's attempts to keep them alive. In future, therefore, society might be forced to adopt a "policy of 'weeding out'" these "degenerates." This might offend peoples' humanitarian sentiments. Nonetheless, he stressed, it was precisely the tendency to "regard all human life as sacred however disabled or worthless or even repellent the individual might be" that had forced society to contemplate euthanasia in the first place.

Like Williams, Joseph Fletcher believed the time had come to jettison conventional "humanitarianism" and define new standards of moral and ethical conduct. Fletcher (1905–1991), born in Newark, New Jersey, was the most important figure in the American right-to-die movement between World War II and the Ronald Reagan presidency. In 1966, he introduced the highly influential theory of "situational ethics," which stated that there were no absolute moral standards that guided medical treatment, and that right and wrong depended upon the particular circumstances facing the individual patient. Fletcher viewed situational ethics as a counterpoint to Catholic literature on the topic, and since the 1960s, no single theory has influenced the field of bioethics more than Fletcher's.

Yet, long before he founded situational ethics, Fletcher had established himself as one of America's best-known secular liberals. When he announced in 1967 that he found Christian doctrine—"God, Jesus, revelation, sin, salvation"—essentially "weird and untenable," it surprised none of the theologians he had been debating for years. Fletcher roundly denounced Catholicism for being "authoritarian" and "alien to our American life and thought where cultural and religious pluralism is the most vital principle."[16] An early supporter of abortion rights, Fletcher had also been active in the family-planning movement and was a friend of birth-control pioneer Margaret Sanger. Fletcher had joined the ESA along with Sanger in the 1940s. His involvement in the Soviet-American Friendship Society prompted Senator Joseph McCarthy to dub Fletcher the "Red Churchman."

Fletcher liked to depict himself as immersed in a titanic struggle to defend democracy and personal, private choice from religious totalitarianism. By eschewing the old-style Darwinism of earlier euthanasia advocates, he often sounded convincing. But a close examination of Fletcher's writings reveals he was as interested in social control as he was in individual choice. Fletcher believed that euthanasia (or "death control") was a kindred cause to reproductive rights for women. "Death control, like birth control," he maintained, "is a matter of human dignity. Without it persons become puppets." To prevent people from becoming puppets, he defended involuntary euthanasia and compulsory sterilization of the handicapped. It was "indecent" for the disabled and terminally ill to go on living, if only because they were "constantly eating up private or public financial resources in violation of the distributive justice owed to others." "The needs of others have a stronger claim upon us morally" than those of individual patients, Fletcher concluded, demonstrating once again how twentieth-century euthanasia activists had trouble limiting mercy killing to just those consenting, dying adults who said they wanted it. Fletcher, echoing earlier euthanasia proponents such as C. Killick Millard and Charles Potter, claimed all ethics were historically contingent and depended on each individual's needs. If that were the case, why not put people whose quality of life appears poor out of their misery, even if they never ask for it? Fletcher could be accused of many things, but never of failing to candidly follow his ideas to their ultimate conclusions.

IMPASSE

Joseph Fletcher and Glanville Williams plainly believed they were fashioning a new, viable, and secular approach to medical ethics as an alternative to Catholic doctrine. But not all early secular bioethicists agreed with them. Their support for legalized euthanasia drew severe criticism from Yale Kamisar, a University of Minnesota law professor. Kamisar agreed with Leo Alexander's "small beginnings" theory and the argument that euthanasia was a slippery slope. A non-Catholic, Kamisar preferred "leav[ing] the religious arguments to the theologians" and instead focused on the civil liberties side of the euthanasia issue. While he doubted that Nazi-like medical murder would ever come to America, he was extremely worried that legalizing euthanasia in the United States might lead to grave abuses. The "legal machinery initially designed to kill those who are a nuisance to themselves may someday engulf those who are a nuisance to others," he warned. It could happen, Kamisar cautioned, if society accepted that there were lives "not worthy to be lived." It was only a small step from there to believing that some people were "better off dead." Euthanasia legalization, he argued, was unnecessary because doctors were getting better and better at controlling pain with medication, and sometimes a misdiagnosis might lead an individual to request aid in dying if it were legal.[17]

Kamisar's forthright interpretation of euthanasia could not have come at a worse time for the euthanasia movement. Struggling to establish its credibility from a bioethical perspective and shake the Nazi stigma, the movement needed all the help it could get. It certainly did not need a legal expert like Kamisar highlighting its similarities to Nazi medical atrocities. In fact, on both sides of the Atlantic, the euthanasia movement entered the 1960s hamstrung by opposition from all of the major churches and medical organizations. To euthanasia sympathizers, the prospect of winning medical and church approval looked as daunting as ever. In the words of Canadian right-to-die activist Olive Ruth Russell, "the stranglehold of tradition and religious dogma" was the most powerful obstacle standing between euthanasia advocates and what she called "the freedom to die."[18]

Yet, no matter how grim the situation looked, hope still lingered within the ranks of the euthanasia movement. Most of its advocates in America and Great Britain had been involved in earlier struggles to win clerical and medical acceptance of birth control. The victories in that endeavor were ample reason to think that similar support would be forthcoming in the future. In the early 1930s, the worldwide Anglican church, the Central Conference of American Rabbis, the Federal Council of

Churches, and (unsurprisingly) the Universalist and Unitarian churches had all sanctioned the use of contraceptives. Surely, euthanasia advocates reasoned, legal euthanasia was just around the corner.

However, resolutely standing in the way of such trends was the Roman Catholic Church. Professing to speak for true Christian values, Catholic officials warned of the "false pity" in which support for euthanasia was wrapped. Even in Great Britain, where they constituted a small segment of the population, Catholics exercised a sturdy influence over public policy through publications such as the *Universe* and the *Catholic Medical Journal*. British Catholics, like their co-religionists in America, warned that there were striking parallels between Nazi practices and what was happening every day to vulnerable patients in English hospitals.

Thus, by the 1960s, it appeared as if an impasse had been reached. Yet, in a few short years, the struggle over euthanasia was about to take a surprising turn. It was about to get more bitter than ever, and it was poised to become an issue of global concern. By the end of the twentieth century, many persons in modern society were not sure exactly what they thought about euthanasia. But virtually no one could say that he or she had never heard of it.

NOTES

1. Henry Friedlander, *The Origins of Nazi Genocide: From Euthanasia to the Final Solution* (Chapel Hill: University of North Carolina Press, 1995).

2. N. D. A. Kemp, *"Merciful Release": The History of the British Euthanasia Movement* (Manchester: Manchester University Press, 2002), 127.

3. Richard Weikart, *From Darwin to Hitler: Evolutionary Ethics, Eugenics, and Racism in Germany* (New York: Palgrave Macmillan, 2004), 215.

4. Kemp, *"Merciful Release,"* 122.

5. Ian Dowbiggin, "'A Prey on Normal People': C. Killick Millard and the Euthanasia Movement in Great Britain, 1930–1955," *Journal of Contemporary History* 36 (2001): 59–85.

6. Kemp, *"Merciful Release,"* 140–141.

7. Stephen Louis Kuepper, "Euthanasia in America, 1890–1960: The Controversy, the Movement, and the Law," Ph.D. dissertation, Rutgers University, 1981, 231.

8. Kuepper, "Euthanasia in America," 95–127.

9. Roy Porter, *The Greatest Benefit to Mankind: A Medical History of Humanity* (New York: Norton, 1998), 656.

10. Ian Dowbiggin, *A Merciful End: The Euthanasia Movement in Modern America* (New York: Oxford University Press, 2003), 85.

11. John T. McGreevy, *Catholicism and American Freedom: A History* (New York: Norton, 2003), 184.

12. Paul Blanshard, *American Freedom and Catholic Power* (Boston: Beacon Press, 1949), 125–127.

13. McGreevy, *Catholicism and American Freedom*, 220.

14. McGreevy, *Catholicism and American Freedom*, 221.

15. Kuepper, "Euthanasia in America," 251–252.

16. McGreevy, *Catholicism and American Freedom*, 250–252.

17. Dowbiggin, *A Merciful End*, 105–106.

18. Dowbiggin, *A Merciful End*, 124.

6

COLLISION COURSE

Despite all the progress made by the euthanasia movement in the twentieth century, by the 1960s it was effectively moribund. The Nazi stigma surrounding the word "euthanasia" showed no signs of lifting. In 1962, when three Germans were tried for their complicity in Nazi Germany's euthanasia program, commentators drew a connection between Nazi medical murder and advocacy of euthanasia in America and Britain. Worldwide, the only two euthanasia advocacy groups were barely surviving. Public support for legalizing euthanasia had flattened after some impressive gains just before World War II. The cultural and political influence of the Roman Catholic Church, a formidable foe of legalized euthanasia, seemed more powerful than ever.

Yet all this was due to change shortly. In the 1960s, death became a topic of vital cultural concern. Greater openness about death shifted attention to the ways people had been dying in recent years, especially the increasing use of intensive, high-technology medical care and the growing numbers of elderly people who were dying in hospitals, rather than at home. The aging of the population in the industrialized world also fueled swelling interest in death as a biological and psychological experience. At the same time, numerous critics charged that organized medicine's attitudes toward the sick and dying were paternalistic and insensitive.

The upshot of this cultural ferment in attitudes toward death was an escalating interest in euthanasia. The heartrending stories of Karen Ann Quinlan and Nancy Cruzan generated widespread sympathy for patients' rights to refuse unwanted treatment, and the ESA and VELS revived their efforts to legalize euthanasia. In the 1970s and 1980s new, grassroots right-to-die groups formed in several countries. The Netherlands emerged as the world leader in tolerating both assisted suicide and mercy killing. The emergence of AIDS in the 1980s likewise boosted support for a right to die. As the twentieth century approached its end, even the most cautious euthanasia advocates were optimistic that the new century would witness the decisive breakthrough they had long awaited.

THE HOSPICE AND PALLIATIVE-CARE MOVEMENT

Yet, well before this critical juncture in the history of euthanasia was reached, the hospice and palliative-care movement arose in the 1950s. Cicely Saunders, a British doctor, former nurse, and student of Christian scholar C. S. Lewis, almost single-handedly launched this campaign in favor of better pain management and spiritual counseling for terminally ill patients. She founded the first modern hospice, St. Christopher's, now a part of the British health-care system. The first American hospice opened in 1974, and by 1982 eight hundred hospice programs were underway in the United States. The number of hospices worldwide has continued to grow, serving hundreds of thousands of patients a year.

Hospice is a throwback to the early medieval concept of a way station for pilgrims and travelers, as well as for the destitute and dying. Saunders viewed hospice care as "a powerful force for undercutting the movement for active euthanasia."[1] She argued that the distress and suffering of the vast majority of dying patients could be treated successfully. If some terminally ill patients requested mercy killing, it was chiefly because modern medicine had neglected their needs, she contended. They were usually anxious due to physical pain and depressed because they felt a severe loss of dignity. Saunders insisted that they would never beg for medical assistance in dying if they were better cared for. Her conclusions have been confirmed by other experts in the field, such as Memorial Sloan-Kettering Cancer Center's Kathleen Foley, who found in her own medical practice that suicide requests "dissolve with adequate control of pain and other symptoms."[2]

Saunders's efforts not only helped to improve a field of health care desperately in need of reform. Her views showed persuasively that relatively simple changes in the way medical personnel dealt with the dying could curtail demand for euthanasia, weakening the rationale for legalized euthanasia. Euthanasia proponents, however, continued to justify physician-assisted suicide by pointing out that better pain management could not relieve the suffering of roughly one in ten terminally ill patients, as Saunders's own studies showed.

THALIDOMIDE

In the 1960s, a new and revolutionary chapter in the history of euthanasia, rivaling the coming of Christianity hundreds of years earlier, was opening, as advocacy of euthanasia was becoming respectable again. One reason was the Thalidomide tragedy. Thalidomide, a drug originally developed in West Germany, was used in the late 1950s by pregnant women both as a sedative and to combat severe morning sickness. It was considered so safe that it was available without prescription in some countries. But it rapidly became a horror story that raised many of the same issues as Harry Haiselden's decision in 1915 not to provide surgery that would prolong the life of a baby born deformed and with serious medical complications.

By the time Thalidomide was finally withdrawn from the market in 1961, its use had accounted for between 8,000 and 9,000 babies born worldwide with severe physical deformities. Thalidomide had never been approved for use in America, but about 500 Thalidomide babies were born in England. It was in Belgium, however, that the Thalidomide tragedy dovetailed most closely with the history of euthanasia. There, in 1962, the parents of a Thalidomide baby were acquitted of murdering their daughter. The case generated enormous press coverage, and newspapers were flooded with readers' letters expressing deep sympathy for the parents. Suzanne Vandeput, the mother, told the media: "I knew I could not let a baby live like that. . . . If only she had been mentally abnormal. . . . She would not have known her fate. But she had a normal brain. She would have known."

Commentators tended to agree with Vandeput, repeatedly questioning what quality of life Thalidomide babies would enjoy. Some, like Brock Chisholm, a Canadian and the first director general of the World Health Organization (1948–1952), advocated euthanasia for such unfortunate human beings. As the VELS noted, this case "brought home to very many people all over the world the whole problem in a way that had not happened before."[3] The VELS never explained why the relatively small number of Thalidomide children caused this media firestorm, when the thousands of disabled babies born every year in England and America did not. But there is no mistaking VELS jubilation that the euthanasia debate was back on the front pages of newspapers around the world.

POPULATION CONTROL

The comments of figures such as Brock Chisholm about the impact of Thalidomide and an increasing concern about global population growth helped to stimulate interest in euthanasia. Chisholm was just one of numerous opinion-makers on the world scene who warned about the dire social, economic, military, and environmental consequences of high fertility rates, especially in developing countries. World population had reached the billion mark in 1750 and quickly shot up to 2.5 billion in 1950. Demographers predicted that the rising population would produce mass famine, enormous environmental pollution, and world war as heavily armed nations would resort to militarism to grab their share of the earth's dwindling resources. Echoing the alarmism that surrounded much Cold War rhetoric, experts argued that population growth caused political instability, which in turn left some nations susceptible to communist takeover. As Chisholm contended, population pressure would breed "hopelessness," paving the way for the "present flight to authoritarianism."

With the stakes of population growth so high, activists felt justified in advocating extreme measures to curb global birthrates. The Canadian euthanasia supporter Olive Ruth Russell urged mercy killing to deal with "the surging rise in the number of physically and mentally crippled children" caused by the "population explosion." Henry Van Dusen, ESA member and former president of the Union Theological Seminary, committed suicide with his wife in 1975 when both were in failing health. They concurred that there was no dignity in living any more under increasing medical care, but they also stated that in a world of rapid population growth, declining space, and too many mouths to feed, their continued existence just wasted precious resources.

Two of America's foremost population-control proponents were backers of euthanasia. John D. Rockefeller 3rd, founder of the Population Council and an avid defender of gay and abortion rights, also devoted considerable time and money to advocating the mass use of contraceptives in poor and populous countries such as India. Just before his death in 1978, Rockefeller had demonstrated a dawning interest in funding groups that endorsed active euthanasia for people with disabilities. Hugh Moore, inventor of the Dixie Cup, was less polished and more prone than Rockefeller to outspokenness on population issues, but he, too, used his immense wealth to spread the message that the global birthrate had to be drastically reduced. Moore coined the term "the population bomb" years before biologist Paul Ehrlich popularized it in his 1968 best-seller of the same name. While Rockefeller accepted all forms of contraception, Moore particularly promoted the use of vasectomy for men and tubal ligation for women as birth-control methods, hinting broadly that compulsory sterilization might be necessary if family planning programs did not sharply curb global fertility soon.

In the 1960s, Moore and his followers dominated the Manhattan-based Association for Voluntary Sterilization (AVS), a group that tried to widen access to sterilization services in hospitals and clinics in the United States and overseas. The link between euthanasia and population control was especially evident in the ranks of the AVS, many of whose members also belonged to the ESA, including Margaret Sanger, Alan Guttmacher, and Joseph Fletcher. Moore eventually left one-quarter of his estate to the Euthanasia Educational Council, the ESA's successor organization.[4]

Most proponents of population control realized euthanasia was too controversial as a means of easing population growth. The strongest affinity between activists of both causes was the belief that the Cold War world was fraught with grave challenges to the very existence of the human species. Many euthanasia and population-control activists, like the environmentalists who began organizing in the 1960s and 1970s, maintained that only a radically new system of values could save the globe from destruction. In a seemingly overcrowded world, people could hardly expect to have as many children as they desired. Similarly, the traditional idea that each individual life was sacred appeared outdated when the populations of countries such as India and China were nudging close to the billion mark. A new system of values that granted people the right to say how, when, and where they died seemed to make eminent sense to many people in the 1960s. Yet, amid the anxious rhetoric of impending global catastrophe, it sometimes sounded as though this freedom was more a duty than a right.

PIUS XII

Given the Roman Catholic Church's opposition to legalizing mercy killing, it was ironic that no one was more responsible for thrusting the topic of euthanasia into the spotlight again than Pope Pius XII (1876–1958). Nearing the end of a turbulent papacy that spanned World War II and the early Cold War, Pius stated in a 1957 address to an international gathering of anesthesiologists that a doctor was obliged only to supply "ordinary" treatment to seriously ill patients who were "deeply unconscious." "Extraordinary" treatment included artificial respiration. As long as the unconscious patient's prior wish to die was known and he or she was "of age," the doctor was not bound to attempt resuscitation if doing so proved to be a "burden" on the patient's family. To Pius, it was no sin for doctors to let nature take its course under these circumstances.

These and other remarks uttered by Pius XII in 1957 about medical care for the dying did not signal an abrupt departure from traditional Catholic teaching about death and dying. But occurring when they did, they helped to alter the entire debate over euthanasia. For millions around the world, his comments redefined euthanasia as a process whereby it was morally permissible to withhold unwanted, unnecessary treatment as long as it was clearly the patient's wish. Letting people die rather than killing them mercifully became the new focus of discussion about euthanasia. This sudden change caught euthanasia supporters in the ESA and VELS by surprise. As an ESA member lamented inelegantly in 1962, "we are in the rear of the late Pope." For years, activists had been advocating euthanasia in terms of a doctor's immunity from prosecution for hastening a patient's death through lethal injections, or the state's right to end the lives of handicapped persons whose care and treatment were costly and only prolonged lives of suffering and unproductivity. It was time, a VELS member remarked in 1973, to reframe the discussion of euthanasia in terms of the medical profession's duty to be more responsive to patients' wishes. The debate over euthanasia was about to shift away from a doctor's right to kill to a patient's right to be left alone to die. Although it was not what they wanted, euthanasia advocates gradually viewed this change as an important step toward convincing society that a right to die included a right to medical assistance in dying.

THE GRAYING OF SOCIETY

The redefinition of euthanasia as essentially a passive, patient-centered practice gained credence thanks to remarkable changes in demography and medical technology. By the 1950s, it was hard for opinion-makers such as Pope Pius XII to ignore the unprecedented power of modern medicine to prolong life. Respirators, artificial feeding machines, and kidney dialysis devices were perhaps the best-known of these medical innovations. Antibiotics, too, helped to revolutionize health care by preventing the elderly from dying from pneumonia. In an earlier era, pneumonia had been dubbed "the old man's friend" because of the way it sometimes speedily killed the aged.

In the brave new world of modern medicine, pneumonia ceased being a killer disease.

The grim irony of medical miracles was that more and more people were living longer than ever before, only to succumb to the degenerative diseases of old age. Throughout the twentieth century, life expectancy in the industrialized world rose steeply, leading to an increasing percentage of elderly people in the population. One of the first symptoms of this demographic shift in the United States was the 1958 formation of the American Association of Retired Persons (AARP). Over the next forty years, the AARP steadily grew to become a powerful political lobbying group headquartered in Washington, D.C., and representing about half of all Americans over the age of fifty.

It was not long before government, too, recognized the graying of the American population. As early as 1961, the U.S. Senate formed a permanent Special Committee on Aging (SCA). A dialogue swiftly unfolded about the quality of life for the climbing numbers of elderly persons. U.S. politicians talked about "rights for older Americans," including the right to "retire in health, honor, [and] dignity."[5] Concern for elderly Americans was particularly evident in 1971 during the SCA hearings on "death with dignity." The SCA chair, Senator Frank Church, insisted the hearings were not about euthanasia. Yet they inevitably raised questions about the practice and future of health care for the elderly. A perception was rapidly crystallizing that modern medicine tended to make death undignified.

The lethal, degenerative diseases of the twentieth century that often afflicted the elderly were by no means new, but their incidence was rising alarmingly. Tuberculosis or influenza may have killed their ancestors, but late twentieth-century men and women faced instead the prospect of dying (often slowly) from cancer, stroke, heart disease, or diabetes while modern medicine frantically tried to keep them alive. When these patients were famous people, the news spread around the world. A 1975 United Press Agency report announced that the doctors treating Spanish dictator General Franco on his deathbed "are using everything they have in a determined effort to keep him alive." The eighty-two-year-old Franco was hooked up to at least four separate mechanical devices: one to help him breathe, one to shock his heart back to normal when it slowed or faded, one to help push his blood through his body, and one to clean his blood. That was not counting the tubes used to aid his breathing, drain fluids from his abdomen, and relieve gastric pressure on his digestive tract. "The effort in itself is remarkable," ran the story, "considering he has had three major heart attacks." Such an "undignified" death would have been inconceivable only thirty years earlier.[6]

Euthanasia activists, trying to justify a right to die, eagerly pounced on these tendencies in health care to prolong life at any cost. VELS member and noted English psychiatrist Eliot Slater cited the example of a seventy-six-year-old British woman in poor health who was suddenly felled by a stroke. Paralyzed and unable to speak, she had actually stopped breathing by the time an ambulance had conveyed her to a hospital. But the medical staff in the emergency ward worked furiously to restore her breathing, keeping her on a respirator for eighteen hours until she finally died. When asked why he had tried so hard to keep her alive, the ward physician said he was not trained to ask such questions. His sole duty lay in saving her life no matter what the cost or inconvenience.[7]

To Slater, such cases raised the troubling question of whether the patient's quality of life was enhanced by merely prolonging "the automatic action of heart, lungs, and bowels." Showing his eugenic perspective, Slater insisted that letting her die would have been a "benefit to the race" and would have reduced the "burden on society" to pay for her care. In the next few decades, Slater and other euthanasia proponents would curtail their social and economic justifications of euthanasia. They quickly learned that concerns about medical technology could be exploited for their own ideological purposes.

MEDICAL NEMESIS

The mind-set in organized medicine stressing whatever means possible to ward off death was symptomatic of a "can-do" attitude that pervaded the profession, and it conformed to the cardinal beliefs of twentieth-century organized medicine: (1) that researchers, practitioners, hospitals, and medical schools should run their own affairs as they saw fit; and (2) that the more medicine society received, the healthier it was. Nowhere was this more evident than in surgery, where many medical students were taught "when in doubt, whip it out."[8] In light of the prevailing ethos, it was hardly surprising that rates for unnecessary surgery, such as hysterectomy to remove a healthy uterus, spiraled upward during the 1960s. In 1974, a U.S. Senate investigation disclosed that over 2.4 million unnecessary operations were performed yearly in America, causing 11,900 deaths and costing $3.9 billion. Hospitalization rates likewise soared, despite evidence that many patients fared better on an out-patient basis.

By the early 1970s, the perception was forming that these generous doses of medicine were not actually making people any better. In *Medical*

Nemesis (1975), the Austrian-born, ex–Catholic priest Ivan Illich went so far as to claim that the medical establishment was a threat to public health. Heart transplant surgery, first performed in South Africa by Christian Barnard in 1967, created a worldwide media feeding frenzy, but it also raised the question whether some lives were worth extending even if it were medically possible. Governments could still declare "a war on cancer" in the 1970s, but the public was becoming more and more doubtful that this was a struggle medical science could win. Survival rates for cancer patients increased between the Depression and the 1970s, but a postmodern patient distrustful of organized medicine was emerging. Many of these patients refused to accept what doctors said as the gospel truth and instead educated themselves about health issues. But many other patients tended to interpret bodily sensations as signs of disease rather than just the everyday aches and pains of life. They appeared to be perpetually nervous about their own health and, though generally healthier than their ancestors, incongruously felt worse about their condition.[9]

The fallout from this overmedicalization was what one historian called "the end of the mandate" for organized medicine by the 1970s.[10] In 1952, an American writer had described patients as "completely under the supposedly scientific yoke of modern medicine as any primitive savage is under the superstitious serfdom of the tribal witch doctor."[11] Within a few short years, however, unthinking deference had turned into wary suspicion. Criticism of the profession peaked in the 1970s, especially within the emerging women's rights movement. Denouncing the paternalism of male doctors and the harm done to women by the health-care industry, women's groups demanded the medical profession admit more women into its ranks and called on women to take medicine "into their own hands" through self-medication and improved public education initiatives. This campaign in favor of gender privacy and empowerment led to publications such as *Our Bodies, Ourselves* (1973), a best-selling, self-help manual of women's health.

Complaints from the women's movement were part of a wider therapeutic counterculture that called for a democratization of medical knowledge and denounced professional dominance over the whole field of health care. Countless people opted for self-help strategies or folk or non-Western treatments. By the end of the 1970s, it was clear that the pre-1960s public reputation of doctors was badly frayed. Growing numbers of patients viewed their relationships with their physicians as adversarial rather than cooperative, demanding that doctors pay more attention to patients' own perceptions of their illnesses. "The patient as a whole" became the new mantra of medical reformers.

Adapting to this shift in perception, in 1972 the American Hospital Association issued a Patients' Bill of Rights, including the right to informed consent and to considerate and respectful care. The American Medical Association quickly followed suit, declaring in 1973 that patients needed to agree with the treatment options offered by their physicians. In 1991, the U.S. Congress passed the Patient Self-Determination Act, which ordered all hospitals, hospices, and nursing homes participating in Medicare and Medicaid programs to inform patients of their right to refuse unwanted treatment. Growing recognition of patients as a valid interest group in their own right made it easier and easier to conceive of patients obtaining a right to co-manage their own deaths.

As the pre-1960s confidence that orthodox medicine was always good for society declined in the 1970s, policy-makers increasingly wondered where valuable health-care dollars could be saved. In 1962, the prestigious English medical journal the *Lancet* noted:

> if the average length of a patient's stay in hospital is two weeks, a bed in that hospital occupied by an unconscious patient for a year could have been used by 26 other patients, whose admission has been correspondingly delayed. Apart from the addition to human suffering which this involves, the life of one or more of these 26 could actually have been lost through delay in obtaining necessary treatment. In a country without a surplus of hospital beds, an irrevocably unconscious patient may sometimes be kept alive at the cost of other people's lives.[12]

This triage mentality about rationing health care became even more popular in later years, when health-care spending as a percentage of national GDP rose alarmingly in most industrialized countries. The similarity between anxious post–World War II debates over how to pay for state health-care services and debates in German medicine between the two world wars over whose lives were more worth saving did not escape the notice of euthanasia opponents.

THE DISCOVERY OF DEATH

Alongside the mounting worry about health-care spending priorities, ambivalence about medical authority, and interest in patients' rights was a remarkable upsurge in concern about death. Starting in the late 1950s, the public was deluged by a steady stream of books, films, magazine articles, and radio and television shows on death and dying. Under the ominous shadow of nuclear Armageddon due to the buildup of atomic weapons, a "death craze" swept modern society. In America, books about death were appearing at the rate of about one per month around 1970, prompting one book reviewer to refer to a "death renaissance." Sales for Elisabeth Kübler-Ross's pioneering *On Death and Dying* (1969) quickly approached half a million. Movies such as *Brian's Song, I Never Sang for My Father,* and *All That Jazz* revealed that Hollywood's customary emphasis on sex and violence had broadened to cover death under high-tech, medical auspices. Many viewed this interest in death as a consequence of the 1960s openness about sex. "First it was sex," stated a Michigan physician in 1976, "and now it's death. . . . The 1970s are the age of Thanatology." In the public mind, death was the last taboo. As Eliot Slater asserted, it was time for society to "let some light into [death's] dark cupboard," just as Freud had enlightened people about their "neurotic" attitude toward sex.[13]

All of this translated into a greater collective willingness to talk about death. But once unleashed, this openness frequently transformed itself into a self-indulgent talkativeness that continued to haunt society for decades. Indeed, interest in death led to troubling consequences. Critics warned that Kübler-Ross's theory of a five-step process of dying (denial, anger, bargaining, depression, and acceptance) could easily become the normative way prescribed for *all* people to die. A Thanatology movement took shape, preaching that death was a positive experience that should be celebrated rather than feared or hushed up.

No wonder some observers asked whether the public discussion of death was all that healthy. Some drew a connection between late twentieth-century society, gripped by a seeming obsession about death, and the late Middle Ages, when the popular *ars moriendi* and other cultural products stressed the imminence and grotesque reality of death. Healthy or not, well-intentioned or not, modern society's preoccupation with death had grown so much by the mid-1970s that it could only indirectly be traced to the specific issues raised by changing medical technology. The "death craze," although certainly affected by the new ways of dying created by high-tech medical care, derived from a deep cultural malaise exacerbated by economic inflation, environmental degradation, energy shortages, campus unrest, and the war in Vietnam. Yet it also stemmed from a radical, society-wide revolution in personal values. By the 1970s, the stage was set for a bitter and highly divisive conflict over how modern men and women defined a "good death," a struggle still raging in the twenty-first century.

KAREN ANN QUINLAN

When she headed to a party with friends on the night of April 14, 1975, twenty-one-year-old Karen Ann Quinlan could hardly have known that she was about to become world famous. Later that evening, she fell into a coma at a New Jersey roadside bar, likely because she had been mixing drugs and alcohol. She was still in a coma three months later, when her parents decided to disconnect her from the respirator that had been keeping her alive at a New Jersey hospital.

The ensuing legal wrangle between the Quinlans and the hospital, which opposed their decision, sent shock waves around the world. Millions around the globe followed Karen Ann's story day after day. For countless people, the plight of Karen Ann Quinlan personalized euthanasia in vivid and moving terms. "Karen Condamnée à Vivre (Karen Condemned to Live)," a *France Soir* headline declared. Her pretty face, captured in a widely distributed high school graduation photo, became instantly and universally recognizable.

By the time the New Jersey Supreme Court ruled in the Quinlans' favor on March 31, 1976, hospital staff had weaned Karen Ann off her respirator. She lived without regaining consciousness for another nine years. In the meantime, the world tried to come to terms with the implications of *In re Quinlan*. What made Karen Ann's fate truly revolutionary was the court ruling that said she enjoyed a right to privacy against intrusion by doctors and the state. Though clearly unable to consciously exercise it, from a legal standpoint she possessed a "right to die." How a right to die translated into reality has become the somber question facing society since the New Jersey Supreme Court decision of 1976.

PUBLIC OPINION IN THE 1970s

Karen Ann Quinlan's tale may not have caused a sudden shift in public opinion about euthanasia. Yet, occurring when it did, it helped to crystallize the evolving sentiment in favor of a personal right to control the time, place, and manner of one's death. Even before Karen Ann Quinlan became a household name, public opinion supporting euthanasia had swung significantly upward from its low point in the 1950s. When a series of Gallup polls asked if voluntary euthanasia should be permitted by law if the patient is incurably ill, 36 percent of the respondents answered yes in 1950, 53 percent in 1973, 60 percent in 1977, 65 percent in 1985, and 69 percent in 1990.[14] Approval of a right to request the withdrawal of unwanted treatment rose even higher over the same period. In England, support for voluntary euthanasia also increased in the 1960s and 1970s.

This rising tide of support for euthanasia beginning in the 1960s certainly mirrored the shifting circumstances surrounding death and dying in a highly medicalized society. But survey results look more impressive than they really are. Pollsters are the first to admit that backing for euthanasia declines the more they ask questions that apply to specific medical situations. For example, approval of euthanasia drops sharply for situations in which the patient's and the family's wishes are discounted. Ultimately, polling on euthanasia conforms to the "rule of thirds": one-third of respondents adamantly support legalizing euthanasia, one-third adamantly oppose it, and one-third back it in isolated cases but oppose it under most circumstances.[15]

Additionally, polling may not accurately reflect what the public truly wants its elected representatives to do about euthanasia. In Britain, where public survey findings appeared to condone acts of voluntary euthanasia, there were few signs that the country was ready to endorse its legalization. For example, in 1969 the VELS tried again to introduce a voluntary euthanasia bill in the House of Lords. In the wake of the parliamentary decriminalization of suicide (1961) and therapeutic abortion (1967), VELS hopes were high that the growing acceptance of individual freedom in these areas would translate into tolerance for euthanasia. But the bill was defeated on second reading by a vote of 61 to 40. Typical of the opposition to the bill was a rabbi who asserted: "we cannot agree to purchasing the relief from pain at the cost of life itself.... One of the reasons for our position is that we consider human life to have infinite value and therefore every fraction of human life, even only one hour of it, has precisely the same infinite value as the whole of life."[16] The VELS was encouraged by the forty votes the legislation had garnered. But tempering its satisfaction was the realization that it takes more than favorable poll numbers to legalize euthanasia.

THE EUTHANASIA MOVEMENT REBOUNDS

Between the late 1960s and the 1990s, euthanasia organizations in the United States and Britain experienced a revitalization of sorts. As interest in and sympathy for the various forms of euthanasia mounted, euthanasia group membership grew exponentially and financial contributions multiplied. In Britain, the VELS changed its name to the Voluntary Euthanasia Society (VES) in 1969, and in 1979 it became EXIT. In America, the ESA reconstituted itself as the Euthanasia Educational Fund (EEF) in 1967, the Euthanasia Educational Council (EEC) in 1972, and Concern for Dying (CFD) in 1978.

These name changes were sure signs that the cultural landscape regarding euthanasia was shifting tectonically in the 1970s. They also reflected the attempts of euthanasia groups to adapt to public mores. At one time, ESA officials imagined themselves as opinion-makers. By the 1970s, they realized that public sentiment could not be manipulated so easily. The word "euthanasia," with its sinister overtones of mercy killing or Nazi medical murder, was being supplanted by the concept of a right to die. As advice columnist (and ESA member) "Dear Abby" (Abigail Van Buren) noted in 1974, "a bill with the word 'euthanasia' in it will never get passed."[17] At a time when women, African Americans, Native Americans, homosexuals, and other groups were demanding equal rights, talk of a right to die resonated with millions of people throughout Western society who saw the issue first and foremost as one of personal autonomy.

One sign that the movement was thriving was the public eagerness to discuss euthanasia. A common sight were American and British advocates at euthanasia symposia at hospitals, medical schools, and university campuses. They were aided by American entertainers Arthur Godfrey and Patricia Neal, who publicly endorsed a right to die. As one ESA member later reminisced about the 1960s: "we were so eager to break the barrier of silence surrounding euthanasia [that] some of us would willingly sit up all night to be able to get on talk shows, and would accept any invitations to talk with students and other groups."[18]

THE LIVING WILL

One reform that emerged from the intense public discussion of euthanasia in the 1960s and 1970s was the living will, a legal document that specifies in advance what kind of treatment a dying patient would want. The idea had actually cropped up within ESA ranks back in the 1940s, but euthanasia advocates in those days were far more interested in legalizing mercy killing than making it easier for terminally ill patients to refuse undesired and futile treatment. By the late 1960s, amid the public furor over use of life-prolonging medical machinery, the living will was an idea whose time had come. In 1969, the EEF drafted a model living will and printed 5,000 copies. Within months, all had been distributed. By 1978, about 3 million living wills in total had been distributed by the EEF/EEC (including 600,000 in the nine months after the Quinlan trial). Periodic endorsements from advice columnist "Dear Abby" were a major factor behind the living will's popularity.

In 1976, California became the first state to recognize the living will. By 1990, forty-one states and the District of Columbia had enacted living-will legislation. Millions of Americans wrote their own living wills, but over time it became apparent that the document was no panacea. The living will is "a virtual failure," commented one bioethicist in 2004. "It's very hard for people to predict their preferences for an unknown health condition," another U.S. ethicist added. It proved to be extremely difficult to address all possible end-of-life situations, especially as life-sustaining technology continued to rapidly evolve. Hospitals also found living wills difficult to interpret. When patients, families, and health-care providers disagreed over what living wills meant, litigation was frequently the result. By the end of the twentieth century, ethicists were recommending people make health-care proxy statements or designate someone to make medical decisions for them (durable powers of attorney), rather than rely on a living will.

Some right-to-die activists were not content with the legalization of passive euthanasia. They had their sights on bigger victories. In Florida and Montana, advocates led ultimately unsuccessful attempts to legalize active euthanasia. Governor Tom McCall of Oregon emerged as the politician most closely identified with euthanasia when his sponsorship of right-to-die legislation failed in the state legislature. Nonetheless, McCall's efforts were a harbinger of later events in Oregon. In 1997, Oregon became the first American state to permit physician-assisted suicide.

THE PLEA FOR BENEFICENT EUTHANASIA

In 1973, the American Humanist Association (AHA), founded in 1941 and the descendant of Charles Potter's First Humanist Society of New York, asserted that an individual's "right to die with dignity, euthanasia, and the right to suicide" were fundamental civil liberties. An AHA document read:

> Our customs and laws seem based on either the premise that death is the most terrible thing that can happen, regardless of circumstances, or the premise that our lives belong to a deity who demands every effort to postpone death. The latter, being a religious concept, has no place in the laws of a country having constitutional separation of church and state. Humanists do not place the responsibility for suffering upon a deity, but accept personal responsibility to correct the evils of our society. We value individual freedom, human rights.[19]

One of the AHA's programs was the National Commission for Beneficent Euthanasia (NCBE), formed in 1974 and advocating both active and passive euthanasia. That year, the NCBE issued its "Plea for Beneficent

Euthanasia," which was "an appeal to an enlightened public opinion to transcend traditional taboos" and endorse the legalization of both active euthanasia and letting people die. The plea was signed by prominent figures such as bioethicist Joseph Fletcher, biologist Linus Pauling, and philosopher Sidney Hook.

Historically, the AHA had enjoyed close links to Felix Adler's Ethical Culture. These ties strengthened in the 1960s and 1970s as militant AHA and Ethical Culture support for euthanasia grew. These groups had shed their earlier religious trappings and become outright secular organizations. Their followers preached a purely individualist approach to medical ethics, stripped of any semblance of creed or common doctrine. The fact that the euthanasia cause received robust support from humanist groups in other countries, including England and Australia, confirmed that the intimate association between humanism and euthanasia advocacy was not restricted to America. It also confirmed that the international debate over euthanasia for the rest of the twentieth century had at least one foot firmly planted in the past.

THE EUTHANASIA MOVEMENT GOES INTERNATIONAL

The first signs that the euthanasia movement was becoming truly international surfaced in the 1970s. Groups in Australia and South Africa were formed, joining the existing organizations in Britain and the United States. The World Federation of Right-to-Die Societies was formed in 1980, uniting twenty-seven euthanasia groups from eighteen countries. Officially, the federation agreed that there would be no common program or policy, leaving each group free to pursue its own goals. But as later events would prove, most members of the World Federation were in favor of both the legalization of mercy killing and physician-assisted suicide.

The origins of the World Federation dated back to 1976, when the Japan Euthanasia Society was founded and invited other right-to-die groups to the First International Euthanasia Conference in Tokyo. Delegates from Britain, America, Australia, Japan, and the Netherlands attended the conference and adopted the "Tokyo Declaration," which supported the legal recognition of a person's right to die without suffering. In 1978, a Second International Euthanasia Conference was held at the University of California at San Francisco. Ten delegations from eight countries attended. Two years later, the Third International Euthanasia Conference met in England, where the delegates agreed to establish the World Federation.

A major spokesperson for euthanasia at the San Francisco Conference was Joseph Fletcher. Fletcher had never been completely happy with the way the euthanasia movement (as he put it) had "soft-pedaled" active euthanasia since the early 1960s in an effort to win popular support for passive euthanasia, or letting patients die. That was "old-hat already," he announced in 1973. To Fletcher, the genuine ethical frontier involved decisions by individuals as to when, how, and where they wanted to die. Deciding to die when one was already dying was no ethical decision at all, he argued provocatively. The time had come to move to the next stage of euthanasia activism, advocacy of assisted suicide and active euthanasia. Fletcher's call for a more radical stance antagonized many in the American right-to-die movement, including the more cautious Concern for Dying. But his admonition was actually more faithful to the movement's history than CFD's position, which was mostly dedicated to public education about the medical conditions surrounding death. Fletcher's declaration resounded with other constituencies in other regions of the United States, notably the West Coast. His message resonated most strongly, however, in the Netherlands.

DUTCH EUTHANASIA

During World War II, doctors in the Netherlands had refused to obey orders from their German occupiers to comply with Nazi medical norms. Although some Dutch physicians were arrested and sent to German concentration camps for defying orders to practice medical murder, the country's doctors would not be intimidated. In a stunning example of how defiance of Nazi rule could be successful, the Germans backed down. As psychiatrist Leo Alexander noted after World War II, "if the medical profession of a small nation under the conqueror's heel could resist so effectively, the German medical profession could likewise have resisted had they not taken the fatal first step."[20]

Yet, less than thirty years later, health care for the terminally ill in the Netherlands changed. A nation that only a few years earlier had roundly condemned any propaganda in favor of euthanasia was in the process of launching a massive experiment in death and dying. What happened to bring about this mammoth change? The Netherlands, like other countries, was hit hard by the cultural revolution of the 1960s. But no Western nation embraced the counterculture attack on long-standing norms more than the Dutch. Even the medical profession was swept along by this current. In the words of one Dutch physician, "traditional ethics collapsed in almost every area, including the medical community."[21] Almost overnight, the Dutch adopted the idea that as long as people are going to use drugs, visit bordellos, and conceive babies out of wedlock, the government should regulate these behaviors rather than condemn them. The same thinking applied to euthanasia. Because growing numbers of doctors were helping their patients to die, those who broke the law against euthanasia would not be prosecuted as long as guidelines were followed.

One Dutch physician who approved of euthanasia was Gertrude Postma. In 1973, she was charged with murder for giving her terminally ill mother a lethal injection. After a highly publicized trial, the court found her guilty and gave her a suspended sentence and one year's probation. But the court also effectively struck down the statute forbidding mercy killing, reasoning that the medical consensus should rule, not the law itself. Since then, mercy killing has been permitted in the Netherlands.

The Dutch position regarding euthanasia has been mired in controversy ever since. Throughout the 1990s, studies repeatedly showed that roughly one thousand euthanasia deaths occurred annually without proper patient consent. Approximately 8 percent of all Dutch infant deaths resulted from lethal injections, even though babies obviously cannot ask to be killed. As late as 2001, only about 50 percent of all euthanasia deaths were actually reported, despite the claims of right-to-die proponents who have long argued that making euthanasia legal will make its practice transparent rather than covert. Naturally, doctors in the Netherlands seek to avoid the extensive paperwork involved in officially reporting euthanasia cases. They also dislike having to get a second opinion. And when doctors are caught breaking the law, they are frequently given slap-on-the-wrist sentences.

The worst fears of euthanasia opponents were confirmed in 2003 when a Dutch doctor helped an eighty-six-year-old politician to die. The politician, though in good physical condition, was "tired of life" and killed himself by ingesting a lethal cocktail of drugs. The doctor was tried and convicted, but an appeals court ruled that the doctor had never violated the Dutch law's guidelines. Ultimately, the conviction was upheld by the Netherlands Supreme Court. The Dutch Voluntary Euthanasia Society expressed its disappointment with the higher court decision, indicating that it (like many other right-to-die groups) was not content with the legalization of euthanasia for only terminally ill patients. The Dutch Medical Association demonstrated a similar eagerness to expand the legal definition of euthanasia. In the early twenty-first century, the organization was lobbying for the legalization of nonvoluntary euthanasia. By then, the concept of a right to die was opposed by only a small minority of the country's population. Fears that the growing numbers of Muslim immigrants threatened such Dutch values meant euthanasia was an important issue on the nation's political landscape in the post–September 11 era.

DEREK HUMPHRY AND THE HEMLOCK SOCIETY

As the Dutch gradually decriminalized active euthanasia, events were unfolding across the Channel that would provide a major boost to the international movement in favor of assisted suicide. In 1978, British journalist Derek Humphry and his second wife, Ann Wickett, published *Jean's Way*, a best-selling account of how Humphry had helped his first wife, Jean, commit suicide as she was dying of cancer. The British police ultimately decided not to charge Humphry, but in the meantime he relocated to Los Angeles, where he and Wickett founded the Hemlock Society in 1980. In only a few short years, Hemlock, begun on a shoestring budget and dedicated to the decriminalization of assisted suicide and active voluntary euthanasia, boasted dozens of local chapters across America, tens of thousands of members, and a newsletter whose subscriber list had grown to 40,000 by 1992. Humphry lectured the world over and was a frequent guest on television and radio talk shows.

The Hemlock Society was a grassroots, West Coast organization that broke the Manhattan-based leadership historically exercised by the ESA over the American movement. In the words of one activist, Hemlock's typical supporter was the "little old Ohio lady in tennis shoes." Hemlock radicalized the entire euthanasia movement. Humphry pushed it in a policy direction that the established, moderate euthanasia groups on both sides of the Atlantic Ocean were loath to follow. Since the 1960s, the successor groups to the ESA and VELS had emphasized raising public awareness about death and dying and the promotion of living wills. Humphry and Hemlock wanted to return to the old agenda of the ESA, particularly the legalization of mercy killing. Other euthanasia radicals applauded. In 1989, Joseph Fletcher urged the whole American movement to "go down the road with Hemlock."[22]

Hemlock's stand on assisted suicide was controversial enough, but Humphry seemed congenitally unable to stay out of trouble. Following the example of the Scottish branch of the British right-to-die group EXIT, Humphry published two books in 1981 and 1991 that provided information on how to kill oneself, including correct lethal doses of drugs. Critics attacked Humphry for irresponsibly publishing a "cookbook of death" at a time when about half a million young Americans were known to try suicide every year. Even other euthanasia advocates attacked Humphry for apparently validating people's decisions to end their lives rather than providing them with the full range of information about treatment options.

The event that most tarnished Humphry's reputation as a compassionate advocate of death with dignity was his very public separation from Ann Wickett. Humphry left Wickett in 1989, shortly after she had been diagnosed with breast cancer. According to Wickett, the marriage had been on the rocks since 1986, when Humphry and Wickett had helped her parents die. To this day, questions linger about Humphry's involvement in the double suicide and whether he had browbeaten them into requesting aid in dying. Wickett also alleged that Humphry had actually suffocated Jean to death, not simply supplied her with the drugs to kill herself. In 1991, distraught over Humphry's desertion and her legal wrangles with Hemlock, Wickett committed suicide and left behind a note for Humphry that read: "There. You got what you wanted. Ever since I was diagnosed as having cancer, you have done everything conceivable to precipitate my death." Wickett also wrote an anti-euthanasia activist just before she died that Humphry was "a killer. *I know*."[23] Humphry countered that Wickett suffered from a "borderline personality disorder," but her disturbing accusations hurt the euthanasia cause.

While Humphry and Ann Wickett were building the Hemlock Society from the ground up in America and generating support for assisted suicide, some supporters of euthanasia back in England were becoming more radical. In 1978, Nicholas Reed, a right-to-die firebrand, became the new head of the VES. Two years later, he and another member of the group were convicted of aiding several suicides, including some persons who were alcoholic, depressed, or otherwise mentally ill. Reed was prosecuted because he assisted the suicides of several people whose full ability to consent was questionable. The overall effect of Reed's conviction was to alert the public to the lengths he and other euthanasia activists before and after him were willing to go to change the law.

THE EUTHANASIA MOVEMENT SPLINTERS

The growing internationalization of the euthanasia movement caused problems. For the first time in history, sizable organizational backing for euthanasia was not limited to Britain and the United States. Support for euthanasia was spreading across oceans and was steadily gaining adherents every day. To optimists within the movement, it appeared as if the great turning point in the history of euthanasia had been reached, after which legal acceptance of assisted suicide and mercy killing would simply be a matter of time. But simultaneously, the first significant divisions within the euthanasia movement, especially in the Anglo-American world, were beginning to form. As the movement became increasingly global, pluralism and diversity, once welcomed, subverted organizational unity.

Even in the heady 1970s, cracks had formed in the solidarity of the U.S. euthanasia movement. In earlier days, "the questions of euthanasia seemed much simpler, and the goals far clearer than they do today," an ESA member said from the vantage point of the mid-1970s.[24] Before the breakthrough in the 1960s, it seemed as if the whole world was against them, and euthanasia proponents felt a kinship then that was as comforting as it was deceptive. Once acceptance of the right to die spread, differences about ultimate aims and agendas surfaced with mounting regularity among euthanasia advocates. For example, fault lines began to form between the less radical American group Concern for Dying and right-to-die organizations in other countries. These divisions surfaced most visibly at the 1984 meeting of the World Federation of Right-to-Die Societies in Nice, France, where various speakers strongly endorsed assisted suicide. Many on CFD's board were distinctly uneasy about what the group called "the European view" of advocating "what, in this country and in many others, is clearly 'murder.'"[25]

Concern for Dying also engaged in a bitter battle with the American group Society for the Right to Die (SRD). Both were splinter groups from the original ESA. In 1985, the two organizations settled out of court after a lengthy and acrimonious legal wrangle over a $1 million bequest. In the late 1980s, the two organizations merged, but in the process purged some SRD members (including Joseph Fletcher) who favored legalizing assisted suicide. The unhappy relations between CFD and SRD in the 1970s and 1980s were testimony to the growing divergences over strategy, philosophy, policy, and personality within the widening euthanasia movement.

In the short term, these differences were a nuisance for right-to-die activists, who struggled to exploit the unprecedented popularity of their cause. Of more serious concern were other unfolding developments that by the end of the century would cause no end of trouble for the euthanasia movement, most notably in the United States.

THE RIGHT-TO-LIFE MOVEMENT

Throughout most of the 1960s, the euthanasia movement benefited from the fact that the once militant opposition from the Catholic Church had faltered.

In 1950, the church had appeared to speak with one voice on all issues regarding sex, reproduction, and death. By 1970, Catholic unanimity was a thing of the past. As the aftershocks of the Second Vatican Council (1962–1965) rippled throughout the world, a liberalization of Catholic doctrine and ritual occurred. Amid a general spirit of ecumenical reconciliation with other religions, many Catholics marched arm in arm with others protesting the Vietnam War or supporting civil rights for African Americans. Within the church, reform became the keyword, as Catholics "threw away fish on Friday, liturgical Latin, [and] tough rules for the priests and nuns." "For its pains," lamented Catholic William F. Buckley Jr., editor of the conservative *National Review*, the Vatican "got emptier and emptier churches."[26] The plight of the traditional church was poetically expressed in the title of Garry Wills's book *Bare Ruined Choirs* (1972). The certitudes that had guided the church for centuries were under heavy attack by the early 1970s. Nor did many Catholics, including Wills, think this trend was such a bad thing.

However, the Catholic ship of state steadied somewhat in the 1970s as the abortion issue emerged. Throughout the industrialized world, governments reformed and repealed their abortion laws. Britain liberalized its abortion law in 1967. In Canada, the federal Minister of Justice (and later Prime Minister) Pierre Elliott Trudeau liberalized Canada's laws on abortion and homosexuality, famously remarking that "the state has no place in the bedrooms of the nation." In 1973, the U.S. Supreme Court issued its decision in *Roe v. Wade*, which functioned as a bracing plunge in an icy river for many Catholics the world over. The Court declared that abortion during the first trimester of a pregnancy was a woman's constitutional right akin to the constitutional right to privacy the Court had found in the 1965 *Griswold v. Connecticut* decision. Many Catholics (like Buckley) had not objected to the *Griswold* decision that women enjoyed a right to privacy when it came to contraception. But countless Catholics were appalled by the decriminalization of abortion and vowed to fight it. They swiftly mobilized in America, throwing their weight behind the National Right to Life Committee (NRLC) which, by the mid-1970s, was politically active in almost every state. The NRLC published a torrent of printed material against abortion and enjoyed the financial backing of the United States Catholic Conference. According to one pro-choice activist in 1973, "right to life groups were springing up all over the country. [They are] quite dedicated and mostly Roman Catholic."[27]

For right-to-life groups, it was a short step from opposing abortion to denouncing mercy killing. In 1968, Britain's Catholic press warned that parliament's new abortion law "opened legal and medical doors to a new Bill promoting the legalization of voluntary euthanasia."[28] A deep respect for the sanctity of human life meant that many right-to-life activists saw euthanasia and abortion as similar crimes against innocent life. Indeed, euthanasia ranked second only to abortion within the pro-life movement as a topic of concern.

Right-to-life activists were highly effective at linking euthanasia and abortion. As one American euthanasia supporter complained, the anti-abortion campaigners "hire very attractive and able speakers. I wouldn't mind if they would stick to the abortion issue, but at no extra expense they invariably sneak in the 'euthanasia dig.'"[29] By the late 1970s, the right-to-life movement was resurrecting the old argument used by Catholic spokespersons back in the 1930s that eugenic sterilization, abortion, and euthanasia were all part of the same agenda threatening the moral purity of America. NRLC members, although mostly worried about abortion, also warned about the mounting strength of the euthanasia movement. To the NRLC, euthanasia proponents were "death peddlers" whose "pagan gods of expediency, utilitarianism, materialism and hedonism" put them squarely on a "collision course" with the "Judeo-Christian understanding of the nature and destiny of man."[30] The NRLC preached the "seamless garment" theory that linked abortion and euthanasia as sinister dangers undermining social justice.

Until the late 1970s, the right-to-life movement was mostly Catholic. Then, as the 1980s dawned, Evangelical Christians joined the crusade. Since the 1920s, Evangelicals, heirs to the early twentieth-century Fundamentalist movement, had kept their distance from the political realm. Beginning in the 1960s, the escalating tolerance of abortion, pornography, homosexuality, and the Equal Rights Amendment for women drove them back into the political arena. Evangelists such as Jimmy Swaggart, Pat Robertson, Jerry Falwell, and Tammy and Jim Bakker took to the airwaves and forcefully expressed their opposition to all these trends. "It is time we come together," announced Falwell, "and rise up against the tide of permissiveness and moral decay that is crushing in on our society from every side. America is desperately in need of a divine healing."[31]

When Ronald Reagan was elected president in 1980, the right-to-life movement had a powerful ally in the White House. Reagan appointed as the surgeon general C. Everett Koop, an ardent foe of abortion rights. In ten short years, the right-to-life movement had grown from modest beginnings into a potent political force and formidable foe of the euthanasia movement. What was once a Catholic crusade had broadened, and right-to-die groups were squarely in the right-to-life activists' crosshairs.

THE AIDS EPIDEMIC

The rise of the right-to-life movement was a major obstacle to right-to-die activists. But in the 1980s, the momentum still appeared to be on the side of the euthanasia movement. The AIDS epidemic, seemingly originating in sub-Saharan Africa in the 1970s, triggered fears around the globe that a new plague had struck. It also boosted support for legalizing assisted suicide, particularly in urban localities where homosexual men, originally the main group at risk for AIDS in the industrialized world, tended to cluster. In 1981, AIDS first came to the attention of physicians in the United States, and in 1983 the human immunodeficiency virus (HIV) was discovered. In recent years the projections of mortality due to AIDS have been scaled back, but AIDS sufferers are still expected to number in the millions, with most of these victims coming from Central Africa.

AIDS, unlike the bubonic plague and other epidemics, kills its victims slowly, reducing them to emaciated and grotesque specimens of previously healthy human beings. The prolonged pain, disfigurement, and loss of dignity caused by AIDS triggered intense bonding among gay men, who increasingly viewed themselves as a group apart from the rest of society, facing a different kind of death. As an American gay playwright noted in 1991, "now I am thirty-one and my lover has AIDS. Our friends have AIDS. And we all take care of each other, the less sick caring for the more sick."[32] They also learned how to help each other die. The suicide rate among gay men soared in the 1980s, far outstripping the rate for heterosexual men. In 2000 in the Netherlands, people with AIDS were twelve times more likely to choose euthanasia than the rest of the population. But, as the Maurice Genereux case demonstrated, if suicides are botched, patients can be left severely disabled and even more helpless than before. As AIDS cut its lethal swath through society in the 1980s, organizations sprang up in gay communities providing aid in dying, and gay men flocked to groups such as the Hemlock Society, seeking effective methods for assisted suicide.

NANCY CRUZAN

In 1983, twenty-five-year-old Nancy Cruzan from Missouri crashed her car and was thrown into a nearby ditch. Fifteen minutes after she had stopped breathing, paramedics got her lungs and heart working. But she was left with profound cognitive disability. Disputes soon broke out over what her exact mental abilities were. What was beyond dispute was that, unlike Karen

Ann Quinlan, her accident did not leave her on a respirator. Nor was Nancy Cruzan terminally ill. To continue living, she needed elementary nursing care: food, fluids, warmth, cleaning, and turning so she would not develop bedsores or pneumonia.

Her parents, however, on the advice of the Society for the Right to Die, filed suit to force the hospital where Nancy was being cared for to remove their daughter's food and fluids. A lower circuit court judge agreed with the Cruzans, but the Missouri Department of Health appealed, and the case began to wind its way to the U.S. Supreme Court. Finally, in 1990, the Supreme Court ruled that life support could be withdrawn from incompetent patients only if there was "clear and convincing evidence" that that was indeed what they wanted. The Cruzans went back to court, this time armed with testimony from two of Nancy's co-workers that, were she to ever become comatose, she did not want to continue living. When a judge ruled in favor of the Cruzans, the Missouri Department of Health abandoned the case, and Nancy Cruzan died on December 14, 1990, twelve days after her food and fluids were withdrawn.

However, Nancy's death did not bring closure to the Cruzan household. In 1996, her father, Joe Cruzan, hanged himself in the family carport at the age of sixty-two, tormented to the last by the gut-wrenching decisions he had made about his beloved daughter's fate.[33]

THE OREGON DEATH WITH DIGNITY ACT

In the short term, *Cruzan v. Missouri Department of Health* buoyed hopes among right-to-die supporters in America. Derek Humphry and others believed that the ruling brought the movement one giant step closer to constitutional recognition of a right to assisted suicide. These hopes appeared to come true in 1994, when the Oregon Death with Dignity Act (Ballot Measure 16) was passed by a 51 to 49 percent margin. The Roman Catholic Church had led the anti–Measure 16 cause, pouring millions of dollars into the campaign. There were two keys to the right-to-die victory in Oregon. The first was the neutral position taken by the Oregon Medical Association. The second was the success the right-to-die forces enjoyed in resurrecting the terms of debate used back in the 1930s and 1940s by advocates such as Charles Potter and his Unitarian, First Humanist Society, and Ethical Culture allies. The right-to-die campaign depicted the contest as "a battle between rigid religionists and compassionate rationalists."[34] In a politically liberal state such as Oregon, this rhetoric about euthanasia being a democratic affirmation of personal choice in defiance of religious dogmatism found a receptive audience in the 1990s. When Oregonians began to believe that euthanasia opponents were trying to impose their morality on other Americans, a slim majority sided with the argument for individual autonomy.

The Oregon law was held up in the courts until 1997, when another referendum roundly endorsed the statute. The law restricts euthanasia to physician-assisted suicide and permits doctors to prescribe oral medications to patients who meet the statute's many preconditions. Only the patients themselves are allowed to administer the fatal dose, and two doctors have to agree that patients have no more than six months to live. Counseling is necessary if a doctor believes a patient who requests aid in dying is depressed. Euthanasia advocates believed that the Oregon law represented a significant harbinger of the future, "a good indicator of where America was headed," in the words of one euthanasia activist.[35] But this sentiment proved overly optimistic. The victory in Oregon was followed by referendum defeats in Michigan (1998) and Maine (2000).

JACK KEVORKIAN

The defeat in Michigan of a right-to-die referendum was due in large part to the Jack Kevorkian factor. Kevorkian, a retired pathologist, was catapulted onto the international stage in the 1990s. Nicknamed "Doctor Death," he first came to widespread public notice because of the plight of Janet Adkins, a fifty-four-year-old music teacher and English instructor from Portland, Oregon. Adkins had just been diagnosed with Alzheimer's disease when in early 1990 she saw Kevorkian on the *Donahue* television show voicing his approval of assisted suicide on demand. She also read in *Newsweek* about Kevorkian's "mercitron," a suicide machine that enabled patients to self-inject lethal doses of drugs. In June of that year, she and her husband flew to Michigan to meet Kevorkian, and it was in his rusting Volkswagen van that she died soon thereafter.

By that stage in his career, Kevorkian was a pariah in the eyes of the medical establishment. He believed not only in euthanasia for both mentally competent and incompetent patients, but also medical experiments on dying, condemned prisoners. When the medical profession failed to endorse Kevorkian's views, he reciprocated by dubbing other doctors "hypocritical oafs" for their refusal to break with traditional medical ethics. In his uniquely defiant and caustic way, Kevorkian in the 1990s trained a spotlight on the issue of physician-assisted suicide.[36]

In the wake of Janet Adkins's death in 1990, Michigan's Oakland County charged Kevorkian with first-degree murder. But the judge threw out the case against Kevorkian because Michigan outlawed neither suicide nor assisted suicide. In 1993, however, the state made assisted suicide a felony, setting the stage for a legal odyssey whose twists and turns over the next several years drew enormous media attention. During this period, juries refused to indict Kevorkian on three separate occasions.

However, in the late 1990s, Kevorkian's reputation took a nosedive. Like Humphry and other radical activists before and since, the longer he remained in the limelight, the more his credibility dissipated. As he helped person after person to die, the facts gradually formed a disturbing tale. Of the sixty-nine people Kevorkian helped to die between 1990 and 1998, only seventeen were found to be terminally ill. Many were not in any physical pain. Also troubling was the fact that 71 percent of his victims were women, a striking statistic in light of the fact that suicide rates are lower among women than men. Some journalists alleged that Kevorkian preyed on vulnerable women with serious illnesses.

As the news about Kevorkian's actions circulated in the 1990s, patience with him and his flamboyant attorney, Geoffrey Fieger, wore thin. The brilliant but ruthless, crude, and verbally abusive Fieger persistently echoed the message of other members of the euthanasia movement that the debate over the right to die pitted rationalist defenders of personal liberty against authoritarian religious groups. When a Michigan judge ruled against Kevorkian, Fieger called her "a malignant bigot" and insisted she had no right to "grant injunctions on moral issues."[37] Fieger's propensity for outspokenness rapidly turned him into a public relations nightmare for the right-to-die movement. By the end of the 1990s, Kevorkian, too, looked more and more like a sinister figure haunting the perimeter of accepted medical practice. Kevorkian's heyday was "a defining moment in medicine," proclaimed the American Medical Association's vice president for ethics standards. "If doctors are allowed to kill patients, the doctor-patient relationship will never be the same again."[38]

By the turn of the twenty-first century, a consensus was beginning to take shape, at least in the United States, around the belief that the law against assisted suicide, though far from perfect, was better than the alternative of sanctioning euthanasia. As a veteran observer of the battle over euthanasia noted in 1994, assisting someone to die, no matter how merciful the intent, "should be left a private act, with society able to be called in to judgement when and if the motive should be impugned. This is not a neat and precise system of justice to be sure, but one that continues to afford the least possibility of abuse."[39]

Dogmatists on both sides of the euthanasia debate might disagree with this statement, calling it far too messy a compromise to last for long. Yet it seemed to capture widespread moderate sentiment throughout the United States and other Anglo-American countries.

Nonetheless, as support for assisted suicide ebbed in the English-speaking world, on continental Europe and in a few other locales around the world, the opposite trend was developing. As the twenty-first century opened, countries such as Belgium, Switzerland, and the Netherlands seemed to be spearheading a shift in the direction of making assisted suicide a legal reality. Additionally, as states grappled with the formidable challenges of funding national health-care systems that guaranteed access and afford-ability for their citizens, evidence accumulated that the euthanasia of count-less elderly, severely disabled, or dying patients was occurring in hospitals, hospices, and nursing homes across the globe. A century of intense debate and often acrimonious conflict had done little to settle the euthanasia issue one way or another.

NOTES

1. Derek Humphry and Ann Wickett, *The Right to Die: Understanding Euthana-sia* (London: Bodley Head, 1986), 191.

2. Edward J. Larson and Darrel W. Amundsen, *A Different Death: Euthanasia and the Christian Tradition* (Downers Grove, Ill.: InterVarsity Press, 1998), 189.

3. N. D. A. Kemp, *"Merciful Release": A History of the British Euthanasia Movement* (Manchester: Manchester University Press, 2002), 179.

4. Ian Dowbiggin, " 'A Rational Coalition': Euthanasia, Eugenics, and Birth Control in America, 1940–1970," *Journal of Policy History* 14 (2002): 223–260.

5. Valery Garrett, "The Last Civil Right? Euthanasia Policy and Politics in the United States, 1938–1991," Ph.D. dissertation, University of California at Santa Bar-bara, 1998, 102.

6. Roy Porter, *The Greatest Benefit to Mankind: A Medical History of Humanity* (New York: Norton, 1998), 700.

7. Kemp, *"Merciful Release,"* 170.

8. Melvin Konner, *Becoming a Doctor: A Journey of Initiation in Medical School* (New York: Viking Penguin, 1987), 103.

9. Edward Shorter, *Bedside Manners: The Troubled History of Doctors and Patients* (New York: Viking, 1986), 211–240.

10. Paul Starr, *The Social Transformation of American Medicine* (New York: Basic, 1982), 379–419.

11. John C. Burnham, "American Medicine's Golden Age: What Happened to It?" *Science* 215 (1982): 1474–79, 1475.

12. Kemp, *"Merciful Release,"* 183.

13. Garrett, "The Last Civil Right?" 111–112.

14. Henry R. Glick, *The Right to Die: Policy Innovation and Its Consequences* (New York: Columbia University Press, 1992), 83–87.

15. Ezekiel Emmanuel, "Whose Right to Die?" *Atlantic Monthly*, March 1997, 73–79.

16. Humphry and Wickett, *The Right to Die*, 85.

17. Ian Dowbiggin, *A Merciful End: The Euthanasia Movement in Modern America* (New York: Oxford University Press, 2003), 140.

18. Dowbiggin, *A Merciful End*, 137.

19. Dowbiggin, *A Merciful End*, 128–129.

20. Wesley J. Smith, *Forced Exit: The Slippery Slope from Assisted Suicide to Legalized Murder* (New York: Random, 1997), 91.

21. Smith, *Forced Exit*, 91.

22. Dowbiggin, *A Merciful End*, 157.

23. Rita Marker, *Deadly Compassion: The Death of Ann Humphry and the Case against Euthanasia* (London: HarperCollins, 1993), 230. Wickett's emphasis.

24. Dowbiggin, *A Merciful End*, 137.

25. Dowbiggin, *A Merciful End*, 221.

26. Patrick Allitt, *Catholic Intellectuals and Conservative Politics in America, 1950–1985* (Ithaca: Cornell University Press, 1993), 188.

27. Donald T. Critchlow, *Intended Consequences: Birth Control, Abortion, and the Federal Government in Modern America* (New York: Oxford University Press, 1999), 197.

28. Kemp, *"Merciful Release,"* 192.

29. Dowbiggin, *A Merciful End*, 148.

30. Garrett, "The Last Civil Right?" 222.

31. Peter G. Filene, *In the Arms of Others: A Cultural History of the Right to Die in America* (Chicago: Ivan R. Dee, 1998), 107.

32. Filene, *In the Arms of Others*, 213–214.

33. Filene, *In the Arms of Others*, 168–183.

34. Dowbiggin, *A Merciful End*, 171.

35. Dowbiggin, *A Merciful End*, 174.

36. Sue Woodman, *Last Rights: The Struggle over the Right to Die* (New York: Plenum, 1998), 91.

37. Garrett, "The Last Civil Right?" 218.

38. Filene, *In the Arms of Others*, 191.

39. Dowbiggin, *A Merciful End*, 175.

7

CRADLE AND GRAVE

The twenty-first century had barely started when Unitarian minister George Exoo and Krishna monk Thomas McGurrin arrived in Ireland, looking like nothing more than a couple of typical tourists. However, Exoo and McGurrin were not in Ireland to see the sights. After Exoo returned to the United States, the Irish authorities charged him with assisting the January 25, 2002, suicide of Rosemary Toole-Gilhooley, a forty-nine-year-old Dublin woman. By prosecuting Exoo, Ireland became the first nation in history to seek the extradition of someone to face charges of helping another person die. If convicted, he could face up to fourteen years in prison. Exoo, already suspected of assisting about one hundred other suicides, has never denied he helped Toole-Gilhooley die. He freely admits that he and McGurrin were present when she swallowed crushed pills, covered her head with a plastic bag, and breathed in enough helium to kill twenty people.

The Exoo case at the beginning of the new millennium highlighted many of the old and new themes that already marked the history of euthanasia. The morality of euthanasia, especially in the form of assisted suicide, has long been conflated with the morality of suicide. Exoo is only one in a long line of euthanasia advocates asking why assisted suicide should be against the law. If it is not a crime for people to end their own lives, why is it a crime to help these same persons to die? But critics point to the huge difference between society's consensus that suicide is an unmitigated human misfortune and Exoo's own validation of Toole-Gilhooley's personal choice to request help in killing herself.

Exoo's religious affiliation reflects that, for much of the twentieth century, the Unitarian-Universalist Association was in the forefront of the campaign to legalize euthanasia. Unitarian backing for assisted suicide, made official in 1988, stems from the association's long-standing belief that social values do not derive from a transcendental source of authority but from human beings themselves. Throughout the twentieth century, Unitarians and their allies in Ethical Culture and humanist groups assailed the traditional Judeo-Christian moral codes regarding sex, reproduction, and death. Legal euthanasia, by seemingly freeing individuals from what Margaret Sanger once called the "biological slavery" of dying painfully, was a quintessentially Unitarian cause. Yet, in constructing an argument for an individual's right to die, some Unitarians and other supporters went as far as earlier advocates who claimed that for certain individuals it was indeed *right* to die. To some, assisted suicide became the right thing to do, belying the notion that euthanasia is a straightforward matter of personal choice.

Additionally, by taking a brazen attitude toward laws prohibiting assisted suicide, Exoo was emulating surgeon Harry Haiselden and pathologist Jack Kevorkian. In fact, Exoo invited people in his home area of western Pennsylvania and West Virginia to call him "the local Jack Kevorkian." His intention, like Kevorkian's, has been to commit sensationalist acts that attract widespread media interest in the hopes that legislatures, the courts, and the public would realize the need to legalize euthanasia. Exoo, Kevorkian, and Haiselden dared the authorities to arrest them. They openly described themselves as latter-day John Browns compelled to break laws they considered as unjust as slavery.

Another historical aspect of Exoo's actions had to do with the mental state of Rosemary Toole-Gilhooley. By assisting her suicide, Exoo demonstrated how difficult it was for any act of euthanasia to be purely voluntary. Exoo advertised his services over the Internet, where numerous websites provide information on how to kill oneself, including the site belonging to the sinister Church of Euthanasia. Tragedy often results when troubled persons visit these sites. This is what happened to twenty-one-year-old Julie Veteto of Arkansas, who in 2001 hanged herself from her bathroom doorway with a dog leash after learning how to do it on the Internet. Veteto was fighting severe depression at the time. The Internet likewise brought Rosemary Toole-Gilhooley and Exoo together. She saw his website and contacted him electronically, offering to pay him and McGurrin to come to Ireland to help her die. She was convinced she was suffering from a terminal illness, but the Irish police and her family disagree. They insist that she was not dying and was instead clinically depressed.

The deaths of Julie Veteto and Rosemary Toole-Gilhooley raise the question: can any request for aid in dying ever be truly elective? How can we know if persons like Veteto and Toole-Gilhooley who request assisted suicide are really in their right mind? How free were their choices? Who can ever be sure?

DIVERGING ATTITUDES

If George Exoo's participation in Toole-Gilhooley's suicide underlined many of the long-standing themes of the history of euthanasia in the modern era, it also pointed to key developments that were becoming increasingly evident by the early twenty-first century. For one thing, a gulf in public attitudes toward euthanasia was opening up between continental European and Anglo-American countries. A citizen of Ireland, Rosemary Toole-Gilhooley knew the law there prohibited assisted suicide. But if she had flown to Switzerland, where assisted suicide is legal, she might have been dead within hours of touching down at Zurich airport. She, like seventy-four-year-old Reginald Crew, a retired Liverpool autoworker suffering from a motor-neuron disease, could have taken advantage of Switzerland's liberal euthanasia law. There, the euthanasia group Dignitas might have supplied her with the drugs to kill herself. Crew died from taking a deadly barbiturate the same day in early 2003 he arrived in Zurich. Toole-Gilhooley might have become yet another British "suicide tourist" in Switzerland, which at the time of her death held the dubious distinction of leading the world in the number of assisted suicides.

The international euthanasia movement may have started in England, America, and Germany, but by the turn of the twenty-first century it was stagnating in those countries while making inroads elsewhere. In 2001, while suicide tourists flocked to Switzerland, Belgium passed a law permitting a physician to supply a terminally ill person with the drugs he or she needed to commit suicide. Surveys of Spanish doctors found that six out of ten wanted a similar law in Spain. In the Netherlands, as we have seen, both physician-assisted suicide and voluntary active euthanasia are legal. Dutch youth as young as twelve with parental consent are allowed by law to request a lethal injection. Teenagers sixteen and over do not need parental approval. Nor do patients need to be terminally ill to receive euthanasia. Their suffering does not even have to be physical; it can be solely emotional in nature. Indications were that France would sooner or later follow the example set by Belgium or the Netherlands.

Some support for euthanasia has been found in Colombia. Normally Colombia only makes the news because of its alarming rates of drug-related crime and guerrilla violence. Yet in 1997, Colombia's highest court, considered one of the most liberal in Latin America, decreed that no one would be held criminally responsible for taking the life of terminally ill persons who requested it. The court defined a terminally ill patient as someone suffering from cancer, AIDS, and kidney or liver failure (though not Alzheimer's or Lou Gehrig's disease). However, eighteen months after the court's decision, Colombia's senate rejected the ruling, and euthanasia remained an illegal act.

Reminders of the twentieth-century history of euthanasia have surfaced in the People's Republic of China. Just as euthanasia proponents in the past have often supported eugenics, so in China advocacy of euthanasia is mounting in the shadow of the country's 1995 Eugenics Law, hastily renamed the Maternal and Infant Health Law under a torrent of foreign criticism. As part of its broader state policy of curbing demographic growth and improving the biological quality of the nation's population, estimated in 2000 at 1.3 billion, China's 1995 law stipulates that potential marriage partners must have medical checkups to ensure that neither has any hereditary, venereal, reproductive, or mental disorder. Those deemed "unsuitable for reproduction" can be compelled to undergo forced sterilization or abortion.

Once it became permissible for the Chinese state to intervene in the name of collective fitness, leading health officials began referring to the "zero worth" of defective infants. Euthanasia in the form of infanticide is increasingly hailed as "scientific humanism" that protects Chinese society against the "counter-selective" forces represented by disabled infants. As a fellow of the Chinese Academy of Social Science stated:

> As to those already born and afflicted with severe inherited malformations, such as cretins with a stretched tongue or babies suffering from hydrocephalus, their intelligence is very low and even if they can survive, they will never be able to work and live independently, giving their families endless misfortunes, increasing the burden on society and adversely influencing the quality of the population. Painless euthanasia at the moment that such babies appear to the world, it should be said, is a eugenic measure that will benefit the country and the people.[1]

When the news broke in 1996 of abandoned children being starved to death in Chinese orphanages, officials had to admit that, for years, health-care personnel had been discussing the possibility of selecting the "superior" infants for survival and "discarding" the "inferior." The toll on human life due to the Chinese eugenics law, compulsory abortions, and unreported cases of infanticide stemming from the country's one-child population policy has been severe.² As of 2005, euthanasia was still officially criminalized in China, but trends pointed to a reversal of policy in the coming years.

By contrast, in Germany, where events during Hitler's Third Reich remain fresh in the public mind, euthanasia is banned, and physicians' groups assert "killing does not belong to the duties of a doctor." The prospects for the legalization of either physician-assisted suicide or active euthanasia in Anglo-American nations look almost as dim. In Britain, public opinion seems to favor physician-assisted suicide, but most British nurses are firmly against medically assisted suicide, and the British Medical Association is equally opposed to helping patients die. None of the country's major political parties backs euthanasia legislation.

FATAL MISTAKES

The British euthanasia movement tried and failed to get the British parliament to enact a euthanasia bill in 1936, 1950, 1969, 1985, 1991, and 1994. Each time it appears it gets tantalizingly closer to legislative success. But in 1993, the House of Lords Select Committee on Medical Ethics concluded that the few instances in which some form of euthanasia appeared warranted did not justify "a policy which would have such serious and widespread repercussions." The potential for abuse if assisted suicide were legalized was too high, argued the committee. In light of the committee's conclusions, the chances of the British parliament legalizing assisted suicide, much less mercy killing, appear remote. The news in 2004 that intensive-care patients in British hospitals were routinely misdiagnosed confirmed that it was all too easy to make fatal mistakes when deciding if the critically ill deserved euthanasia. Thus, by the time the new millennium began, British right-to-die activists could be forgiven for pessimistically thinking that victory remained as elusive as ever.

In the United States, the findings of the 1994 New York State Task Force on Life and the Law largely agreed with the conclusions of the House of Lords Select Committee. As Supreme Court Justice Anthony Kennedy remarked in 1997 (citing the New York State Task Force), legal euthanasia will in the long run "diminish choices, not increase them." The U.S. Supreme Court's 1997 ruling backed the task force's findings and denied that there was a constitutional right to die. The court did permit individual states to enact euthanasia laws if they saw fit. But right-to-die advocates have since tried and failed in Michigan, Maine, Wyoming, Vermont, and Hawaii to win legislative approval of assisted suicide. When added to their earlier defeats in Washington State (1991) and California (1992), these setbacks augur poorly for the movement in the early twenty-first century.

The lone exception is Oregon, the only American state to vote in favor of assisted suicide. However, studies of how the Oregon law functions point to a cautionary conclusion. According to some critics, a "culture of silence and secrecy" surrounds the Oregon law.[3] The Oregon Health Division relies entirely on doctors' reporting of cases of euthanasia, and typically only after the fact. The state does not attempt to verify data provided by physicians. If it did, it might discover that, despite its safeguards, abuses still occur involving patients with psychiatric disease who are given lethal prescriptions, as reported to the American Psychiatric Association in 2004. And, according to right-to-die activists, the requirement that two physicians approve of each assisted suicide is no obstacle to arranging one. Barbara Coombs Lee of Compassion in Dying told the *Washington Post* in 1998: "if I get rebuffed by one doctor, I can go to another" to get the necessary signatures.[4] Yet, leading physicians such as Marcia Angell, former executive editor of the *New England Journal of Medicine*, believe Oregon's law is still too restrictive and that too few people are using it.

Studies of the Oregon statute indicate that, where assisted suicide is a legal option, palliative care services are deficient and underutilized. These and other findings warn that right-to-die legislation can lead to a reduction in the quality of health care for society's most vulnerable and needy patients.

END-OF-LIFE CHOICES

A telltale sign of the euthanasia movement's decline in America was the 2003 change in name of the Hemlock Society to End-of-Life Choices. In 2004, End-of-Life Choices merged with Compassion in Dying to form Compassion and Choices. Derek Humphry had stepped down as leader of Hemlock in 1992. By then his very public troubles with Ann Wickett had made him more a liability than an asset to the group. Since his departure from Hemlock, he has concentrated on lecturing, research, and writing about euthanasia. The 2003 name change reflects the mounting recognition among right-to-die groups in the early twenty-first century that advocacy of assisted suicide or voluntary active euthanasia does not resonate with most Americans. The name End-of-Life Choices mirrored the growing emphasis in health-care policy on better pain management and counseling of terminally ill patients and their families about treatment options. When it comes to end-of-life choices, Americans appear to want information, education, and consultation more than legislation.

In other words, as the new century opened, the ESA's old dream was in tatters. To longtime activists such as Humphry, it looked less and less likely that they would see euthanasia legalized. There was always the chance that an additional state would follow Oregon and enact a physician-assisted suicide law. But even if that happened, a stampede of other states in the same direction was distinctly unlikely.

These shifts in America's overall mood regarding euthanasia indicate how marginalized Jack Kevorkian and George Exoo had become. Their grandstanding was both cause and effect of the robust opposition to euthanasia from voters, legislators, and the courts. Their actions reflected their desperation, their own realization that legalized euthanasia was unlikely to be achieved through the normal political and legal channels. Their tactics tended to backfire, because for every individual won over to their way of thinking about death and dying, another two or three were so appalled that they became more firmly than ever anti-euthanasia.

This is essentially the lesson learned by the St. Petersburg, Florida, hard-rock band Hell on Earth. In 2004, the band announced it would let a disabled fan kill himself on stage as a way to promote assisted suicide. The suicide never took place, and many regarded it as little more than a publicity stunt for the band. But the controversy sparked by the band provoked the Florida state legislature into passing a bill that banned suicide as a form of entertainment.

PROVOKING CHANGE

In Canada, right-to-die activists had appeared to be winning the battle of public opinion as the twentieth century came to a close. Suicide had been decriminalized in Canada in 1974. But the country's Criminal Code was amended to outlaw assisted suicide. By the early 1990s, the nation's eyes were on thirty-four-year-old Sue Rodriguez who, after Canada's Supreme Court ruled the country's law against assisted suicide did not violate any of her constitutional rights, publicly announced her wish to find a doctor who would help to kill her before her Lou Gehrig's disease did. John Hofsess, who had founded the Canadian Right-to-Die Society in 1991 to (as he put it) "provoke change" along the lines of Derek Humphry's Hemlock Society, agreed to help Rodriguez find such a doctor if she permitted him to publicize her case. His plan was to dare the government into bringing charges against the physician, and later win a dramatic court victory for the right to assisted suicide.

Yet, Hofsess did not count on Svend Robinson, the first openly gay member of the Canadian parliament. Robinson, eager to exploit the situation for political fame, dissolved Hofsess's pact with Rodriguez and supplied her with a mystery doctor who helped her die in February 1994. "How could charges be brought against a 'mystery physician'?" Hofsess later asked. "We were on a roll when the Rodriguez case began, momentum was building, and we had the makings of a winning team. Then Robinson grabbed the ball and fumbled it. This is a case where a personally ambitious politician betrayed the original purpose of the Rodriguez case and turned it into a mere publicity stunt."[5]

In 1995, the Canadian euthanasia movement suffered another blow. A Senate Committee on Euthanasia and Assisted Suicide voted not to change the status quo on assisted dying, sabotaging a free vote on the issue that had been promised by the federal government.

Additional evidence that Canada is not promising ground for the euthanasia movement was the decision of Canadian courts regarding Saskatchewan farmer Robert Latimer. One morning in 1993, while the rest of the family was away, Latimer carried his twelve-year-old daughter Tracy to the barn. There, he locked her in the family truck, ran a pipe from the exhaust into the truck's cab, turned on the ignition, and closed the barn door. Tracy, born with severe cerebral palsy, was dead within minutes. Latimer was later convicted of second-degree murder and sentenced to jail for life with no chance of parole for ten years. Latimer appealed, but in 2001 the Supreme Court of Canada upheld his sentence. The verdict in the Latimer case stands in stark contrast to the lenient manner in which courts historically have dealt with parents who killed their disabled children. The Latimer decision may signal a shift, at least in North America, toward stiffer judicial treatment of individuals who normally have faced sympathetic juries. If so, his case will be a milestone in the history of euthanasia.

Another milestone in the history of euthanasia took place in Australia in 1995, but it proved to be a fleeting victory for the right-to-die forces. That year Australia's most remote region, the Northern Territory, enacted an assisted-suicide law. There had been euthanasia groups in Victoria and New South Wales since the 1970s, when Australian humanist groups had followed the example of their U.S. counterparts and advocated changing the laws prohibiting assisted suicide and voluntary euthanasia. By the 1990s, Australian approval of a right to die had reached the 70 percent mark. At the time the Northern Territory's law was repealed in 1997, Australia was the only place on earth where people enjoyed a legal right to assistance in dying. Australians such as the noted right-to-die activist physician Philip Nitschke hoped that it would be landmark legislation and a turning point in the history of euthanasia. But in retrospect, it may well have been the only victory for the right-to-die movement in that country for a long time.

In the first place, the Northern Territory's statute became law by only a slim 13–12 margin. It was viewed widely as a tribute to the outgoing, popular chief minister of the region rather than a strong statement of principle. Many Australians also worried that the Northern Territory would become the "killing capital of the world." These reasons, coupled with the opposition it sparked from Australian doctors and religious groups, led to the law's repeal in 1997 at the federal level. In 2002, the Australian Medical Association rejected a proposal to soften its stance against euthanasia.

In the meantime, Philip Nitschke has joined Exoo and other activists in designing devices for those who want to commit suicide. Like Exoo, Nitschke also advertises on the Internet. In 2003, Nitschke shifted his main attention from Australia to neighboring New Zealand, opening a branch of his pro-euthanasia group Exit in Wellington. New Zealand's center-left-dominated parliament narrowly defeated a bill in 2003 that would have legalized assisted suicide, and Nitschke believes that the chances of a legislative breakthrough are greater there than in Australia. But his willingness to break the law reflects a dawning realization that the laws banning assisted suicide are not likely to change anytime soon in the rest of the Anglo-American world.

DEMOGRAPHIC CHANGES

What accounts for the differences over euthanasia between continental Europe and the rest of the Western world? One important reason is the widespread secularization that Europe underwent over the course of the twentieth century.[6] It is no accident that the popularity of legal euthanasia spread in countries such as the Netherlands, one of the world's most secular and socially permissive nations. Indeed, rates of Christian churchgoing and self-identification across much of the continent have been dropping steadily for decades, at least among European whites.

However, worldwide demographic currents have been slowing the progress of secularization. Significantly, it is in nations with large immigrant populations, such as Canada and the United States, that the euthanasia movement has slowed to a crawl. Already the homes of robust right-to-life movements, both nations are increasingly attracting deeply religious immigrants from the developing world whose social conservatism rivals that of the most traditionalist Christians. The 1965 Immigration Act continues to reshape the religious complexion of the United States. For example, Latinos, most of whom are Roman Catholics, form one-third of the population of Texas. By 2010, they are predicted to constitute a majority in California. Twenty-five percent of all births in America are of Asian and Hispanic ancestry. Roughly forty-five percent of the population of Toronto, Canada's largest city, is foreign born. Many of these immigrants to North America are Christian, while some are Muslim, Hindu, Buddhist, and Sikh. They tend to be highly religious and opposed to the secular value systems they encounter in their adopted countries.

The same can be said for Britain, where the empire has been striking back in dramatic fashion. By 2003, although the percentage of third-world newcomers within England's overall population remained modest, the majority population of an urban center such as London was on the verge of becoming nonwhite. Whites will likely be in the minority in Britain by the end of the twenty-first century.

In industrialized nations, the influx of ardently religious newcomers conflicts with the secular, rights-based values that normally undergird support for euthanasia. The global reshuffling of people between developed and developing worlds means the other major world religions are exerting more and more influence over the current euthanasia debate in nations where Christians have long predominated. It is surely no coincidence that, in the Netherlands, a vociferous anti-immigrant movement has played an increasingly important role in social policy-making. Before his assassination in 2002, the colorful demagogue Pim Fortuyn had mobilized many voters behind his call for sharp reductions in the admission of newcomers, especially Muslims, to the Netherlands. At the time of Fortuyn's murder, immigrants, many of them Muslims from North Africa and Turkey, formed ten percent of Holland's population. Fortuyn's followers fear that their secularist and individualist values are threatened by an influx of third-world immigrants who likely do not appreciate Dutch policies, including euthanasia, same-sex marriage, government-regulated prostitution, and legal hashish and marijuana use. The 2004 brutal murder of the brash artist Theo Van Gogh (a descendant of painter Vincent Van Gogh) at the hands of a fundamentalist Muslim unleashed ethnic violence in the Netherlands, including attacks against Islamic mosques and schools. Van Gogh's murder rekindled interest in curbing Muslim immigration.

Yet, even if the Netherlands closed its borders, the country may not be able to withstand other demographic forces already underway. Some argue that Western society appears to be heading in the opposite direction from secularization.[7] They assert that the demise of secularism in Western countries is accelerating and that its defenders may be losing the battle for the cradle, especially in the United States. There, the 44 percent of the population that calls itself "born again" tends to favor a family size of three or more children. Evangelicals, along with their allies in other conservative Christian churches, have higher birthrates than parishioners at more liberal churches, such as the Presbyterian, Episcopal, and United churches.[8] By the early twenty-first century, the numbers were beginning to affect polling on euthanasia in America. As the *Chicago Sun-Times* reported in 2003, backing for physician-assisted suicide was ebbing, after decades of rising support. Almost 50 percent of those polled by Gallup said that they thought physician-assisted suicide was "wrong." There may soon be a return to the situation some fifteen hundred years ago when the major organized religions dominated attitudes toward euthanasia.

Still, the ebb and flow of secularization alone cannot account for the fortunes of the euthanasia movement. In the United States, a further irony is that, while euthanasia crusaders such as Kevorkian and Exoo imagine themselves engaged in a struggle akin to the civil rights movement, African Americans tend to be highly suspicious about efforts to overturn the nation's laws against euthanasia. U.S. blacks tend to be poorer, sicker, and have less health insurance coverage than whites. Fifty percent of all AIDS deaths in the United States are African American. The widespread belief is that in a country where the poor often do not have medical insurance, African Americans will suffer disproportionately if euthanasia is legalized. Many U.S. blacks think this is precisely why white law-makers want euthanasia legalized. They are wrong to think so, but the fact remains that some African Americans fear that the efforts of right-to-die groups mask white plans for genocide.

Constituencies that ordinarily might have been sympathetic to euthanasia have also been declaring their stalwart opposition in recent years. Disability activists, including the group Not Dead Yet (NDY), militantly have fought the right-to-die movement. Formed in 1996, shortly after Jack Kevorkian was acquitted of assisting the suicides of two women with nonterminal illnesses, the group has picketed the Hemlock Society's headquarters in the past. Eleven other national disability-rights groups have joined NDY in opposing assisted suicide. Since many of NDY's members are secular liberals who also endorse abortion rights, their very visible opposition to legalized euthanasia signals that not all adversaries of euthanasia are right-wing Christian reactionaries.

OUTLOOK IN THE TWENTY-FIRST CENTURY

If little likelihood existed that either assisted suicide or active euthanasia would be legalized in Anglo-American countries in the early twenty-first century, other forms of euthanasia were being practiced there and elsewhere with distressing regularity. In 2004, British police in Leeds, Hampshire, and Derby were investigating charges that elderly hospital patients were the victims of "mass euthanasia." Hospital staff were alleged to have hastened the deaths of numerous patients by starvation. That same year, local health authorities in Besançon, France, uncovered evidence of at least eighteen cases of mercy killing at the city's University Hospital. The patients included an elderly man in a coma, a man with a self-inflicted gunshot wound to the face, and a victim of a car crash. In some cases, patients were injected with curare, potassium chloride, or a strong mixture of sedatives and painkillers. Nurses and paramedics at the hospital complained that decisions leading to patients' deaths were sometimes made by single doctors without consulting others, including patients' families.

The spirit of Harry Haiselden is alive and well. Every day in hospitals around the world, doctors order nurses to starve defective neonates to death, even in cases where a condition is remedial, as in spina bifida. In the Netherlands, about 8 percent of all infants who die are being killed by doctors. Some bioethicists, such as Princeton University's Peter Singer, justify infanticide. A member of the British Medical Association's ethics committee argued in 2004 that there was no difference between aborting defective unborn children (an accepted practice) and killing babies with defects soon after birth. He insisted that the ultimate decision must lie with the parents, but he did not appear concerned that his line of thinking might lead to infanticide for purely cosmetic reasons, such as nothing more than a cleft palate.

Perhaps the most glaring aspect of the early twenty-first-century debate over what constitutes a good death is that it is so often characterized by historical amnesia. The debate continues to rage as if euthanasia only recently became an issue. Yet, as this book demonstrates, the history of euthanasia stretches back many centuries. Much of the language used to describe death and dying has changed over time, but in many other respects, society is still arguing over basically the same issues. Every day countless judgments about the advisability of keeping certain individuals alive are being made in both clinical and nonclinical settings. Many of these cases involve intensely personal opinions about what is and is not normal medical treatment and when it is time, with death approaching, to let go of life. Bioethicists Peter Singer and Helga Kuhse contend that, because "no one really believes that all human life is of equal value," the time has come to reconsider long-standing ethical attitudes toward life and death. Singer defends the position that some lives are not worth living. Roughly a century ago, Karl Binding and Alfred Hoche said virtually the same thing. Singer's words remind us that today's debate over euthanasia is firmly rooted in the past. His comments, and the historical memories they evoke, also caution us that the global struggle over how society defines a right to die is far from over.

NOTES

1. Frank Dikötter, *Imperfect Conceptions* (New York: Columbia University Press), 160–161.

2. Dikötter, *Imperfect Conceptions*.

3. N. Gregory Hamilton, "Oregon's Culture of Silence," in *The Case against Assisted Suicide: For the Right to End-of-Life Care*, ed. Kathleen Foley and Herbert Hendin (Baltimore: Johns Hopkins University Press, 2002), 175–191.

4. Hamilton, "Oregon's Culture of Silence," 148.

5. Sue Woodman, *Last Rights: The Struggle over the Right to Die* (New York: Plenum, 1998), 133–134.

6. Philip Jenkins, *The Next Christendom: The Coming of Global Christianity* (New York: Oxford University Press, 2002), 94.

7. Jenkins, *The Next Christendom*, 94–99.

8. Philip Longman, *The Empty Cradle: How Falling Birthrates Threaten World Prosperity and What to Do about It* (New York: Basic, 2004).

INDEX

ABOUT THE AUTHOR

Ian Dowbiggin is chair of the history department at the University of Prince Edward Island. He has also taught history at the University of Toronto, Brown University, the University of Dallas, and the University of Rochester. An internationally acclaimed historian, he is the author of four other books on the history of medicine. He was a finalist for the Canadian Historical Association's Wallace Ferguson Book Prize in 2003 for his *A Merciful End: The Euthanasia Movement in Modern America*. A frequent commentator on current events and medical issues, he has been featured on C-SPAN's Book TV and National Public Radio. He serves on the editorial board of the *History of Psychiatry*. He, his wife, Christine, and their children, Beth and Christopher, live in Cornwall, Prince Edward Island.